D0403333

The Heart of a Champion

*My 37-Year War
Against Heart Disease*

Glenn "Bo" Schembechler

Fritz Seyferth

Kim A. Eagle, M.D.

All inquiries should be addressed to:
Ann Arbor Media Group LLC
2500 S. State Street
Ann Arbor, MI 48104

Printed and bound in the United States of America.

1 2 3 4 5 6 7 8 9 10

Library of Congress Cataloging-in-Publication Data.
Schembechler, Bo. The heart of a champion : my 37-year war against heart disease / Glenn "Bo" Schembechler, Fritz Seyferth, [and] Kim A. Eagle.
    p. cm.
    Includes index.
    ISBN-13: 978-1-58726-495-5 (hardcover trade : alk. paper)
    ISBN-10: 1-58726-495-1 (hardcover trade : alk. paper)
    ISBN-13: 978-1-58726-494-8 (hardcover proprietary : alk. paper)
    ISBN-10: 1-58726-494-3 (hardcover proprietary : alk. paper)
1. Schembechler, Bo—Health. 2. Coronary heart disease—Patients—Michigan—Biography. 3. Football coaches—Michigan—Biography.
I. Seyferth, Fritz. II. Eagle, Kim A. III. Title.
    RC685.C6S283 2007
    362.196'1230092--dc22
    [B]
                                                    2007036592

For corporate and bulk sales,
contact bulksales@annarbormediagroup.com
for pricing and availability.

Contents

Foreword

If I were asked to sum up Bo Schembechler in a single sentence, it might be this:

He lived by his heart, and he died by it, too.

Bo knew his fate. He told me so himself. One time, when we were working on his autobiography, he said to me, quite out of the blue, "I will die one day from a bad heart."

It is not the kind of sentence most men utter. Bo was not most men. He was as strong, as direct, and as honest as a human being can be; he could not help but be the same with his mortality.

So he accepted that his heart would beat him at some point, but only in the way he accepted that the clock in a football game eventually shrinks to zero. That doesn't mean you can't fight, kick, scramble, run, push, pull, and bull your way to the last second. And Bo did. He actually, his doctors might tell you, snuck time back onto the clock more than once.

And got away with it.

Why not? He loved life. He honored it. He lived it to his fullest—even though, at the tender age of 40, he suffered his first heart attack, while walking up a hill the night before the Rose Bowl.

He grabbed onto a tree when the pain struck him. He held himself up. And at that moment, he said to himself, "What the hell is happening?"

You could say he spent the next 37 years trying to answer that question.

Bo became a heart expert. He dissected medical information the way he dissected game film. He wanted to know it all. He wanted to know what the doctors knew and what they didn't know. He wanted the latest developments. I'm not sure Bo ever felt he could beat his weak heart. But he sure as heck was going to know its history and its tendencies, just as he would those of an opposing team.

Knowledge, Bo believed, could keep you in a game. And—despite the fact that he snuck a few too many steaks and hamburgers for a man with his health issues—he believed knowledge could keep him alive.

It is fitting that Bo's name is now on a book that examines heart disease. It was always the shadow opponent in his life, the one you didn't read about, the one he was always playing and fighting. In these pages, you will find Bo's heart from the inside and the outside. You will see it as the organ that fought to keep his blood pumping and as the source of his caring personality that made so many players say they loved him and made his funeral and memorial services more like well-attended conventions.

One day, if we are lucky, science will find a cure for the disease that took Bo from us too soon. And at that moment, old coach Schembechler will have won his fight.

Because we can't wait to forget about heart disease. But we will never—and never want to—forget Bo.

—Mitch Albom
Author of *Tuesdays with Morrie* and
For One More Day
Detroit, Michigan, 2007

Introduction

Bo Schembechler had his first heart attack when he was in Pasadena preparing his team for the Rose Bowl, on December 31, 1969. Nearly four decades later, after battling high blood pressure, diabetes, kidney disease, and undergoing multiple cardiac operations, he continued to challenge and motivate all with whom he came in touch across the country—former players, friends, public audiences, and the by-chance acquaintance—to help them realize their potential, just as he had in so many ways.

How could this possibly be? We all know that heart disease and diabetes are progressive, relentless disorders that take the lives of those they afflict long before four decades have passed, right? Well, maybe not. This is the story of how one man, facing tremendous odds, succeeded against a seemingly invincible foe.

Bo spent the last decades of his life counseling others who had cardiovascular disease, giving his advice and support. For this reason Bo wanted this story told. He was always a teacher helping others. His desire was to have this book help all who find that they have cardiovascular disease fight it. Bo Schembechler's medical story is as inspiring as his football legend. But, as you shall see, they are connected.

—Dr. Kim Eagle and Fritz Seyferth

Timeline of Bo's Life and His Fight with Cardiovascular Disease

Date	Bo's Life	His Fight with CVD
April 1, 1929	Bo is born in Barberton, Ohio	
1947–51	Bo attends Miami University and plays football for Sid Gilman as a freshman, George Blackburn as a sophomore, and Woody Hayes as junior and senior.	
1951	Graduate assistant coach to Woody Hayes at Ohio State	
1952–53	Drafted into the Army	
1953–54	Takes first coaching job at Presbyterian College	
1955	Assistant coach to Doyt Perry at Bowling Green	
1956–57	Assistant coach to Ara Parseghian at Northwestern University	
1958–63	Assistant coach to Woody Hayes at OSU	
1964–68	Head coach at Miami University	
1969–89	Head coach at University of Michigan	
1969		Suffers 1st heart attack the day before his first Rose Bowl
1976		First bypass surgery—Quadruple
1986		Diabetes is diagnosed
1987		Second heart attack and second bypass surgery

Date	Bo's Life	His Fight with CVD
1988–89	Athletic Director and football coach at University of Michigan	
1990	President of the Detroit Tigers	
1991	Millie dies of adrenal cancer	
1991	Bo is fired as Detroit Tigers' president	
1992	Bo starts Millie Schembechler Adrenal Cancer Research Fund	
1993	Bo marries Cathy	
2000	Millie Schembechler Adrenal Cancer Research Fund reaches $5 million goal	
2001		Heart failure diagnosed
2002		Neuropathy from diabetes begins
?		Arrhythmia begins (atrial flutter)
2004		Ablation procedure
2004	Bo discusses initiating $10 million Heart of a Champion Fund for CVD research	
2004		First pacemaker is implanted.
2006		Pacemaker/defibrillator is implanted.
November 17, 2006		Bo passes from a heart that just cannot go anymore.

Fast Forward—
1970 Rose Bowl

Bo's story is like so many of each of our stories. It starts with the surprise that we have cardiovascular disease, though the signs that have suddenly come to our attention arrive after many years of progressive disease development. No one was more surprised than Bo when he was told he had had a heart attack! He was doing what he loved to do—staying active, working with young people, and generally living life as he felt it was meant to be lived.

Bo's first heart attack was a lucky wake-up call, for it gave him a chance to learn and grow from the experience. While he may not have stayed true to the heart healthy disciplines in the early years, the lessons learned after that first incident set the foundation for change that enabled Bo to fight his cardiovascular disease so effectively.

Here is how it all started, from Bo's awareness of his cardiovascular disease and his insight on his first heart attack, December 31, 1969.

Bo: I had the traditional symptoms of a heart attack—heaviness in my left chest and an ache going down my arm. What really threw me was I knew something was wrong, but they took me down to a hospital near the Rose Bowl and we took an electrocardiogram ... and nothing showed up!

I found out that a heart attack doesn't necessarily show on the electrocardiogram immediately after the attack. I had a heart attack! I absolutely had the heart attack the day before game day when they hospitalized me. I felt strongly that I had it that prior day, but when they took a look at the electrocardiogram, it didn't show anything, and so I went home and ate a hamburger!

The day before the Rose Bowl game, I knew something wasn't right at football practice. We were practicing in the south end of the Rose Bowl, doing situational plays, different down and distance, at different locations on the field. I was upset with myself and my lack of intensity and focus, so I ran that ball from spot to spot on the field for each of the situational plays. I was thinking, "What is wrong with you? This is the biggest game of your life, and you are not mentally or physically ready!" I couldn't get up for the game. Something's wrong if you can't get up for your first Rose Bowl, the biggest game of your life!

I walked into our equipment room before practice and there were three or four of our coaches just exhausted and laid out in there. They were getting a nap and I remember telling them, "What is wrong with you!? Every one of us needs to be on our game to have this team ready to play. These players need all the motivation we have to give them. We don't have time to feel sorry for ourselves!"

I was pushing myself and everyone else. After that practice, where I ran from spot to spot setting up the next play, we went up to the Monastery. We ate dinner, and the priests wanted me to come down to join them for their New Year's Eve party. I didn't feel like going down there, because I knew I had to come back up the hill and I did not feel well. But I went down and joined the priests. I drank a 7-Up; I thought maybe that would settle my stomach. I was thinking, "Maybe this is indigestion and this is going to settle." I did not stay very long, because word came down that the president of the university had shown up at the Monastery and they wanted me to come up and introduce him to the squad.

So I started up the hill, but I couldn't make it! I got to this big tree and leaned against that tree, and … ohhh, man! I got this sharp pain in my chest. So I stayed there for a while, and when it settled down I went up to introduce President Fleming. I don't know what I said, but I introduced the president and sat down.

Afterward, our Athletic Director Don Canham came over to me and said he thought I was really short with the president because I didn't give him a long enough introduction! But that is all I had in me at that time. I just wanted to sit down.

That night I went around to every player, as I did the night before every game, but I didn't stay as long as I usually did. I wanted to get to bed early. I was exhausted. My discomfort was a dull feeling; I just felt blah. What really got me were not the actual pain and the discomfort, but that I could not shake this lethargic feeling I had.

The day before the Rose Bowl Game I'd had the electrocardiogram and then ate the hamburger and I still didn't feel good. So the coaches came around to see me late that evening after I had checked in all the players. They always did that, and we used to sit and talk last-minute stuff, just trying to capture any final thoughts we may have. I said, "Hey, I'm kind of tired tonight, let's knock it off." So they knew something was wrong and they left.

Then early the next morning, I stayed in bed and tried to sleep. I don't know how. I don't think that I slept real well, but I think I slept some. Then the next morning, Dr.

O'Connor and Dr. Anderson showed up, and they said, "Bo, the way things are going we ought to take another electrocardiogram, and there is a hospital nearby." I went down there and was met by a doctor by the name of Haskell Weinstein. Nice guy. So, I'm lying on the table after they had taken the electrocardiogram, and I'm studying my game plan for the game in a few hours. I had all I needed to win the game on those sheets of paper and I'm studying them, reading, concentrating on the plays, and Dr. Weinstein comes in and says, "Coach, I'm afraid you're out of the game. You've had a heart attack." I said, "Naw, that can't be, I mean No! I mean ... what!?? ..." So I called my defensive coordinator Jim Young to come see me. They gave me a little time with him, because it was Jim Young I wanted to take over the team.

So I told Dr. Weinstein, "Sedate me fast, because I don't want to think about this." I didn't know a single thing about that game until it was over. I didn't know what happened, nobody was bringing me scores, or anything like that. I just laid there in intensive care.

There was no question that I was in the right place after I got the news. It would be like a guy going into a fight when he knows damn well he's not in any shape to win. I knew I wasn't up to it. I could have been tough and stood on the sideline, but I probably would not be here today if I did.

Gary Moeller, Bo's former assistant coach, remembers the night before the game: "Bo said, 'Well you know, I'm really kind of tired tonight. Hey, hit that light when you go out.' And you know, in a very nice way, so I guess he was saying, 'Go if you want to leave; if you don't, we'll sit around, we'll BS a little bit more,' but I said, 'Nah, I'm getting out of here.' So I turned off the light and went out.

Then the next morning he saw Dr. Anderson and they took him to the hospital. He never made it back for breakfast; he didn't make the team meal at all."

That was the end of Bo's first Rose Bowl.

Bo's passion for excellence and attention to detail was communicated to his first Michigan team early, and when he was late for the Rose Bowl team meeting, the team knew something was wrong.

Fritz Seyferth, fullback on the 1969–1971 University of Michigan teams recalls that Thursday morning: "In Bo's first year he started most of our team meetings five minutes early … At our first team meeting with Bo he told us, 'You have to understand that this watch (pointing to his watch as he said it), this watch of mine may not be right. My suggestion is that you be in your seat five minutes early.' So we always showed up five minutes before the start of a meeting. Well, at 11:25, five minutes before the biggest pregame meeting of our lives, Bo is not there, and at 11:30 he's still not there. Then at 11:40 he's still not there, and everyone is wondering, 'What is going on?' Something's wrong, and then Coach Young came in and said, 'Bo won't be with us today.' And I can tell you, we thought there is only one way he is not with us: he's not alive.

"It wasn't until the second half of the game that we found out from a manager who had gone over to the stands to get a ball that had been kicked in the stands. He came back and said, 'They're telling me in the stands that Bo is in the hospital. He had a heart attack.' That's when we learned what had happened."

The development of coronary heart disease is a chronic process, with its earliest manifestation beginning in childhood. The fatty streaks that ultimately become cholesterol-rich plaques on the lining of coronary arteries can be seen in teenagers and young adults. Under the influence of genetic factors and their interaction with risk factors including smoking, high blood pressure, obesity, diabetes, poor diet, sedentary lifestyle, and elevated cholesterol, these coronary plaques may grow and ultimately become vulnerable to plaque rupture with associated heart attack and even sudden death. While Bo Schembechler's first heart attack seemingly came out of the blue, it didn't. It came after years of gradual and very silent disease development.

My Preseason—Age 0–39

As researchers have learned, there are two components that determine cardiovascular health:

1. The genetic makeup inherited from our parents and
2. the lifestyle choices we make.

Bo learned this after his heart attack, as he began to study his family's health history and to reflect on how he had lived those first 39 years. Knowledge is powerful, and it made Bo even more effective in living the balance of his life.

Bo: My problem didn't begin with the heart attack in 1969. Many people look at it that way, but I don't think it begins there. It began with the way I lived my life prior to the heart attack. Going morning, noon, and night, recruiting and traveling all over, stopping for hamburgers at 10, 11 o'clock at night, eating chili on the way home, and pushing myself seven days a week. I mean the pressure and challenges of the new job at Michigan and the Miami of Ohio job before Michigan were immense. Then, it finally caught up with me in Pasadena. Now that's the way I look at it. So actually, it started with how I lived my life up until that time.

Mary Passink, who has worked for the Athletic Department since 1979 and was Bo's assistant from 1998 to 2006, describes him at the office: "When people sent pictures from back in his coaching days to have him sign, he would always say, 'Look how big I was.' You know, you don't remember until you see it in a picture how big he was. But, he worked 18-hour days, he ate on the run. I remember he always did take a nap though, every day, 12:30 to 1:00 every afternoon he was in his La-Z-Boy in his office. He'd close the door, and you didn't dare go in there, unless it was an emergency. And, of course, in those days, he didn't exercise either. He didn't have time."

Lynn Koch, who worked with Bo as his secretary and then assistant from 1969 to 1989, was always "amazed at how long he worked. He'd be in there at 6 o'clock in the morning, and stay until 11 o'clock at night."

Coronary Heart Disease

How is it that Bo Schembechler suffered a heart attack at the young age of 40 years? The answer is that over a number of years, his personal characteristics, health conditions, and lifestyle habits contributed to his developing coronary heart disease. These are called coronary risk factors. It took Bo a number of years to learn that risk factors do more than contribute to initial heart problems. They also increase the chances that existing coronary disease will worsen. When his first heart attack occurred, far less was known about controlling risk factors than we know today.

Certain risk factors, such as getting older, can't be changed. Starting at age 45, a man's risk of heart disease begins to rise, while a woman's risk begins to increase at age 55. But some men and women develop symptomatic heart disease at an even younger age. A family history of early heart attacks or strokes is another risk factor that can't be changed. Bo's father died at a young age of cardio-vascular disease. He succumbed to a stroke. Thus, his family history may have been part of the explanation for Bo's problems at such a young age. Genes may convey risk, but certain families also share other factors such as obesity, a high-fat diet, smoking, and even a sedentary lifestyle.

While some risk factors can't be changed, it's important to realize that patients like Bo have control over many of them. Regardless of age or family history, or how serious their heart disease is, most patients can take steps to reduce their risk of a first or repeat heart attack. Also, working closely with their care team, they can usually successfully manage other problems associated with heart disease, such as angina, heart failure, and arrhythmias (cardiac pulse irregularities).

Once a patient fully understands their coronary risk factors, it is critical that they work hard to address each one. Each risk factor contributes to the progression of heart and vascular disease, so the more risk factors one has, the higher the risk. Risk factors tend to magnify each other's effects. Since Bo had an unfavorable family history, elevated cholesterol, diabetes, and hypertension, not to mention a poor diet, his multiple risk factors made his future problems many fold greater than they would have been if he'd had just a single risk factor.

Bo: Back then, we didn't know as much as we do now. We talked about high cholesterol but there was not much to do for it other than diet. At that time, I wasn't exercising regularly, and my diet was pretty bad. However, I didn't have diabetes yet, and I never did smoke or drink much at all.

I guess that I should have expected to develop heart disease. My sister Marge was 13 months older than I was and she had heart problems. She had a heart attack, but she was getting along real well, got up to retirement, and then she got pulmonary hypertension. Maybe she was in her fifties? She died when she was 72. Marge and I were very close; I loved that girl. She was great, and boy do I miss her.

I was told that, hereditarily, I did not have big arteries. I had small arteries. Now, if you have small arteries, and then you have occlusions besides, that's not good, because you can stand some narrowing if you have nice big fat arteries. That could have been my Dad's problem. He died very suddenly of a stroke. It had nothing to do with the heart. But they say the two problems are related.

The motivation to change today's habits can come with seeing a future, in which you want to play a role, that may not be possible without change. Bo used this thought process to motivate him to change his habits as his cardiovascular disease and related health problems became a more formidable opponent.

In Mary Passink's opinion, "I think his dad and Shemy were always in the back of his mind. I really think he thought a lot about his dad dying at a relatively young age and his son Shemy being so young. He was thinking, 'Am I going to be there when Shemy grows up?' because his dad died in his fifties."

Smoking

Smoking is the "leading cause of preventable death in the United States," according to the Centers for Disease Control and Prevention. If one has coronary heart disease and continues to smoke, the risk of having a heart attack is doubled compared to patients who stop smoking. If a person lives or works with smokers, secondhand smoke can also cause numerous health problems, including a higher risk of heart attack—even if they don't smoke themselves.

Smoking stresses the heart in several ways. The nicotine in cigarettes constricts the coronary arteries, raises the heart rate and blood pressure forcing the heart to work harder than it would otherwise, and tends to lower the good HDL cholesterol. Smoking reduces oxygen levels in the blood. Thus, smoking both increases the heart's need for oxygen and restricts the amount of oxygen it receives. Smoking is associated with heart attacks at a much earlier age because of its effects on the coronary arteries.

Remarkably, cessation of smoking can rapidly reduce the risk of a first heart attack or a second or third one. After just a few days, the blood pressure goes down and the levels of oxygen return to normal. Within one year after quitting, coronary blood flow and breathing are improved. Wisely, smoking was never an issue with Bo Schembechler. If it had been, it seems very unlikely that he would have lived for much longer after his first heart attack.

Bo: I never smoked a cigarette in my life. Every once in a while I would have a cigar, but I never smoked cigarettes, and I was never much of a drinker.

Diabetes and Woody Hayes

Diabetes is a disease about which Bo knew quite a bit because his mentor Woody Hayes had it, and he thought he understood it. They talked about it, and even argued about it. Perhaps as much as anything, it was Bo's understanding of diabetes and Woody's failure to treat his diabetes with the discipline Bo felt he should that upset Bo most about Woody. So when Bo found out he had diabetes, he already was emotionally aware of the implications that came with not taking this disease seriously.

Bo: I found out that I had diabetes in 1986. It was a shock because there was no diabetes in my family ... I mean none. So I had what was described as type 2 diabetes, and I took these pills for a long period of time. Then my cardiologist sent me up to a diabetes expert and I started to work with him. He knew when he came up with shots, I was not coming back. I was not ready for that. He stepped up with that shot and I was saying, "Double my pills if you want, but don't give me that damn shot." He said, "Well, you will only be good so long, and then you've got to take them." So then I relented and started to take shots.

You know, Woody Hayes had diabetes, too. I'm not sure that he had it when I was there, but I only knew later in life he was diabetic.

And, of course, the big thing was that Dr. Bob Murphy, the Ohio State University team physician, felt that the episode in Jacksonville when he punched an opposing team's player during the Gator Bowl game was a result of him failing to take his insulin. They say you can act pretty crazy if your blood sugar is sky-high. Knowing how that works, I can see how that happened if you don't take your shot and it's hot in Jacksonville. The game is going on, it's a close game, and all of a sudden you are going to lose. I don't think that would have happened if he'd taken his insulin.

I remember being in a restaurant with Woody, and he'd sit there and look at a piece of pie. He'd say, "I know

I shouldn't eat it." I said, "Well, then, don't eat it." Then Woody said, "Oh, God damn it, one piece of pie isn't going to hurt you." Then he'd eat it!

He didn't have the same discipline with foods that I have now. We had a reunion, at the University of Miami, Ohio, of the 1950 team. The 1950 team was Woody's last team there. That's the one that beat Cincinnati and went to the Salad Bowl, and did all those things. That was one of his absolute favorite teams, because he knew that team got him the Ohio State job. So, Woody is deadly sick and he made up his mind he was coming to that reunion, and his doctor came with him. He would not miss being with that team for anything.

Then I remember the day before he died he was asked to introduce me at a Kiwanis dinner in Dayton, Ohio. So, he shows up, and he's using a walker. He can barely make it, and his voice is not good, and he comes walking in there, and I was upset. I said, "Why, why would you have him come down here? This is not right." His friends said, "We told him not to come, we told him, and he refused." He had said to me earlier, "I will be there." And so he came.

Well, he got up there to introduce me and actually ended up making a speech. He spoke for a half hour, and you know, he was terrific. And nobody knew at the time this is the last time you are ever going to hear this man. It's over after that. And I have on my desk a tape that some guy took from out in the audience of Woody talking about me and my relationship with him. Boy, it was really good, and it meant a great deal to me.

Woody could barely move at 78, but then he didn't take care of himself at all. Now, he didn't drink, he didn't smoke. He didn't do either of those, but he didn't take care of himself. His diabetes was poorly controlled.

Understanding Diabetes

Patients with diabetes have about the same risk for a heart attack as someone who has already had a heart attack but doesn't have diabetes. Patients with coronary heart disease *and* diabetes, like Bo, have an even higher risk for heart attack than those who have either heart disease or diabetes alone. Up to 75 percent of those people who have diabetes will die of cardiovascular disease, especially following a heart attack or stroke. Diabetes is associated with less successful coronary angioplasty and bypass graft surgery and increases the risk of developing congestive heart failure.

The type of diabetes that most commonly develops in adulthood is called type 2 diabetes, which Bo had and which affected Woody Hayes. In type 2 diabetes, the pancreas makes insulin but the body can't use it properly (known as insulin resistance). So the pancreas produces more and more insulin until it is burned out and no longer able to produce it. Diabetes increases the risk for heart attack, kidney failure, blindness, and peripheral vascular disease, which can lead to leg pain when walking (claudication) and even lower-limb amputation. Diabetes can also lead to nerve damage (neuropathy), difficulties in fighting infection, and delayed wound healing. Despite excellent blood sugar control, Bo suffered from claudication as well as kidney and neuropathic consequences of type 2 diabetes.

The major risk factor for type 2 diabetes is obesity, especially having extra weight around the waist. Most people with diabetes don't know they have it until it is discovered during a routine visit to the doctor that includes a blood sugar test.

Controlling the blood glucose (blood sugar) levels helps to prevent complications. For diabetics, tight control of other risk factors is equally critical. The blood pressure target for diabetics is less than 130/80 mmHg. Managing cholesterol or blood fat levels, avoiding tobacco, and performing regular exercise are all very important. Bo achieved all of these goals with the right medications and disciplined lifestyle.

A Simple Approach to Diabetes Control

For diabetics, five goals are equally important and the patient must be a full and knowledgeable partner in this matter. The first is a diet that is tailored to ideal weight, helps lower the blood sugar, and is high in fiber, beans, fruits, and vegetables and low in saturated fats (found in fatty meats and dairy products) and trans-fats (as in margarine, crackers, and cookies). It often takes a few visits with a dietitian to understand how to shop, prepare foods, eat out, and limit calories to accomplish weight loss.

The second goal is regular exercise that helps lower the blood sugar and improves each of the coronary risk factors. This should be at least 150 minutes a week, about 30 minutes 5 to 6 days a week, equivalent to a brisk walk or about 10,000 steps a day.

The third is to personally monitor the blood sugar at least once and sometimes several times a day depending on the beginning blood sugar and treatments being followed. Another essential measure of blood sugar control is a test called hemoglobin A_1C. This helps one determine how well the blood sugar has been controlled over the last month or so.

A fourth key goal for diabetics is effective blood pressure control. The higher the blood pressure, the harder the heart has to work and the more damage done to the heart muscle, blood vessels, and kidneys. Patients with hypertension or diabetes should measure and keep a blood pressure diary at home. For people with diabetes, we want to keep the blood pressure below 130/80 mmHg. It usually takes at least one medicine to control the blood pressure to the right target, but most patients actually need two to four medication types to control hypertension. Bo checked his blood pressure almost every day. This allowed him to be *sure* that this silent risk factor was not contributing to his risk of future problems.

The fifth key goal for people with diabetes is cholesterol control. LDL, or "bad" cholesterol, builds up and clogs the arteries. LDL cholesterol should be tested at least once a year. The goal is to keep this below 100 mg/dL and usually with a cholesterol-lowering drug known as a statin. In a patient with both diabetes and coronary heart disease, the doctor often advises to aim for a lower target number, for example, less than 70 to 80 mg/dL. High triglycerides and low HDL cholesterol are very common in diabetics, and both increase the risk of progression of vascular disease and heart attacks. Each can be helped by diet, weight control, and exercise and other medications if necessary.

High Blood Cholesterol

We take for granted the statin drugs available to us today, but they were not always available to serve patients in need. Once again, Bo was blessed to ride the wave of medical advancements in cardiovascular disease. As his cholesterol was becoming a greater issue in his cardiovascular health, the statins came on the scene to help him in this battle. Likewise with blood pressure control medications, they were providing critical benefits to patients when Bo needed the help.

Bo: I remember when this disease got my attention in a serious manner, I said, "What the hell happened here? Why did I have a heart attack at 40?" It was obvious that the artery occlusions in there had to be caused by cholesterol, so we've got to do something about cholesterol. I don't remember what the first pill we started taking for my cholesterol was—it may have been lovastatin or simvastatin—but I remember that my cholesterol used to be high, but we didn't have really good drugs for it until the 1980s or so. Remember, my first heart attack was in 1969! But in the 1980s, the statin drugs came out and Rudy Reichert, my cardiologist, put me on one right away. Since then, my cholesterol has been much lower but I've had to change medicines a few times because some of them made my muscles ache.

The higher the blood cholesterol level, the greater the risk of having a heart attack and stroke. If a person has already experienced coronary heart disease, the heart attack risk is higher in persons with high cholesterol. If one has diabetes as well as heart disease, the heart attack risk rises even further. With both diseases, it is extremely important to take steps to keep both the cholesterol and diabetes under tight control. Lowering cholesterol in people with heart disease reduces the need for angioplasty (a catheter to open a blocked artery) and bypass surgery and the risks for future heart attacks, strokes, and death by about 25 to 35 percent for each.

How Does Cholesterol Cause Heart Disease?

The body actually needs cholesterol to function normally. However, the body makes all the cholesterol it needs. Over years, extra cholesterol and fat circulating in the blood can build up in the inner lining of the arteries that supply blood to the heart (called the coronary arteries). This plaque buildup may cause an artery to narrow severely. If enough oxygen-rich blood cannot reach areas of the heart muscle, then chest pain (angina) may occur. If the blood supply to a segment of the heart is suddenly and completely cut off by a blood clot overlying a coronary plaque, then the result may be a heart attack. This usually happens when a soft cholesterol-rich plaque erodes and then a blood clot forms over this area of erosion.

What Kinds of Cholesterol Are There?

Cholesterol circulates in the blood in different "packages" of fat (lipid) and protein, called lipoproteins. Cholesterol that is connected with low-density lipoprotein (LDL) is called *bad* (or *l*ousy, *l*ethal) cholesterol, because a high level of LDL in the blood promotes formation and growth of cholesterol plaques in the arteries. Another type of cholesterol is called high-density (HDL), known as *good* (or *h*appy, *h*ealthy) cholesterol. HDL helps to remove cholesterol from the body, preventing it from building up in the arteries.

Like high blood pressure, high blood cholesterol does not cause symptoms, so when the cholesterol level is too high, people are often unaware of it. This explains why it is important to get cholesterol levels checked regularly, especially if one has heart disease. A blood test called a "lipoprotein profile" or "lipid profile" measures the levels of all types of lipids, or fats, in the blood.

The total cholesterol (TC) is a measure of the cholesterol in all of the lipoproteins, including the bad LDL cholesterol and the good HDL cholesterol. The *higher* the LDL, the greater the risk of heart disease and heart attack. Knowing the LDL number is especially important because it is the first consideration in designing lifestyle and medication treatment to lower cholesterol levels.

Evaluating the HDL level is just the opposite. The *lower* the HDL number, the higher the risk of heart disease and heart attack. An HDL cholesterol level of less than 40 mg/dL is a major risk factor for heart disease and heart attack. An HDL level of 60 mg/dL or higher is protective against heart attack.

The lipoprotein profile blood test also measures the level of triglycerides, another fatty substance in the blood. The target goal for triglycerides is currently less than 150 mg/dL.

The main goal of cholesterol-lowering treatment is to reduce the LDL cholesterol level enough to reduce the risk of heart attack. Achieving this level of control is particularly important if one already had heart disease like Bo. The higher the heart attack risk, the lower the LDL goal is. For most patients like Coach Schembechler, or those with coronary disease and diabetes, the goal of cholesterol-lowering treatment is an LDL level below 100 mg/dL and preferably below 70 mg/dL. Recent medical studies show a direct relationship between lower LDL cholesterol and a reduced risk for heart attack. Doctors now prescribe intensive cholesterol-lowering treatment for people at very high risk for a heart attack. Patients with heart disease and diabetes, or those who have just had a heart attack, often have their LDL goal level lowered by their doctors to less than 70 to 80 mg/dL.

There are two main ways to lower the LDL cholesterol: lifestyle alone or lifestyle combined with medications.

Lifestyle

Effective lifestyle changes to lower LDL cholesterol start with choosing foods low in saturated and trans-fatty acids (the main culprits that raise blood cholesterol) as well as low in dietary cholesterol. Saturated fat is found in fatty meats, chicken and turkey skin, butter and whole milk dairy products, as well as in tropical oils. Trans-fatty acids are created in the process of hydrogenation. Dietary cholesterol is found in all animal foods and is most concentrated in eggs and organ meats such as liver.

LDL cholesterol–lowering works especially well in low saturated-fat diets rich in soluble fiber from oats, dried beans and peas, fruits and vegetables. Heart healthy eating includes at least three servings of whole grains per day, lots of nonstarchy vegetables and fruits, two to three servings of low-fat dairy products, dried beans and peas, small amounts of nuts and seeds, and five to eight ounces of lean meat per day. A heart healthy lunch or dinner may therefore consist of about half a plate of nonstarchy vegetables; one-fourth of the plate with broiled, grilled, or baked fish, chicken or turkey without skin, or beef or pork loin or round cuts, wild meats such as venison or concentrated plant protein such as beans or tofu; and one-fourth of the plate would be whole grains, whole grain products, or starchy vegetables. On the side would be a small helping of fruit and a glass of 1 percent or less milk or a serving of yogurt.

The focus on nonstarchy vegetables and smaller portions of the more calorie-dense meats and starches helps individuals fill up on lots of nutrition with fewer calories. This leads to reaching and maintaining a healthy weight, and healthy weight maintenance, in turn, further helps lower LDL cholesterol. Maintaining a healthy weight and getting regular exercise are especially important for preventing progression of heart disease as well as controlling diabetes. Patients like Bo, who needed to lower LDL cholesterol, benefit greatly from this approach.

Lifestyle Combined with Medications

If the LDL level remains above the goal, then doctors usually prescribe medications known as statins to augment the effects of a healthy lifestyle. It is important to remember that dietary and drug treatments are complementary methods to lower LDL cholesterol and heart attack risk. Taking a medication does not lessen the importance of following a heart healthy diet.

High Blood Pressure

High blood pressure, or hypertension, is another major risk factor for heart disease, heart attack, and stroke. For patients like Bo Schembechler, where heart disease was already present, high blood pressure raises heart attack risk even higher. Hypertension also raises the risks of congestive heart failure and kidney disease, both of which Bo had experienced. High blood pressure is the number one risk factor for stroke, which claimed his father's life.

Blood pressure is the amount of force exerted by the blood against the walls of the arteries. Everyone has to have some amount of blood pressure so that blood can get to all of the body's organs—like water through the pipes at home. Blood pressure is usually expressed as two numbers, such as 120/80, and is measured in millimeters of mercury (mmHg).

The first number is the systolic blood pressure, which reflects the amount of force produced on the arteries when the heart beats. The second number, or diastolic blood pressure, is the pressure that exists in the arteries between heartbeats. The higher the blood pressure, the harder the heart has to work and the more wear and tear on both the heart muscle and on the blood vessels.

High blood pressure is a "silent" killer because it usually doesn't cause symptoms. Thus, many patients with hypertension don't even know that they have it, and many who have recognized hypertension do not control it well.

What Constitutes High Blood Pressure?

The blood pressure category is determined by the higher number of either the systolic or the diastolic measurement. For example, if the systolic number is 115 but the diastolic number is 85, the correct category is prehypertension.

	Systolic		**Diastolic**
Normal blood pressure	Less than 120	and	Less than 80
Prehypertension	120–139	or	80–89
State I Hypertension	140 or higher	or	90 or higher
State II Hypertension	160 or higher	or	100 or higher

High blood pressure is almost always controllable with proper monitoring and treatment. For most patients, blood pressure is considered high when it stays at or above 140/90 over a period of time. However, for patients like Bo who also had diabetes, it is important to keep the blood pressure below 130/80 mmHg. Bo checked and charted his blood pressure nearly every day. This created the opportunity to adjust his treatment week to week rather than simply relying on his regular doctor visits to document his level of control.

Bo was successful in controlling his blood pressure in part by achieving an effective lifestyle. This included keeping his weight down to a near ideal level, regular exercise, reducing salt in his diet, and trying to eat properly. The dietary approach to stopping hypertension (the so-called DASH diet) is rich in fruits, vegetables, whole-grain foods, beans and nuts, and low-fat dairy products. It typically has plenty of magnesium, potassium, calcium, protein, and fiber, but is limited in saturated, trans, and total fat. Bo also strived to limit sweets, sugar-containing beverages, and red meat in his diet.

Unfortunately, for most patients with hypertension, the blood pressure remains high even after lifestyle changes. Depending on the situation, the doctor may prescribe medications from the start, along with changes in lifestyle. There are several different classes of medications that can be used to control high blood pressure. Most patients require two or even three agents, in addition to lifestyle, to achieve consistently good blood pressure control. The strategies of lifestyle and drug treatment are complementary. Thus, more success with lifestyle treatment generally helps to reduce either the number or dosages of blood pressure medications that a patient needs. Bo needed three or four classes of blood pressure medications for a number of years. By using these consistently, he reduced his risk of stroke, heart failure, heart attack, and kidney failure.

The First Quarter—
1969–1976

There was no question that Bo's first heart attack scared him and was his wake-up call. But like so many of us, he lost the discipline needed to fight it as effectively as he could have over time. Initially, we are not aware of cardiovascular disease because it progresses so slowly. We do not feel it until it is critical and, likewise, once the "critical" situation seems to be passing, it is easy for us to revert back to some of our behaviors that got us into trouble in the first place. Cardiovascular disease, once present, is ready to grow as the foods and the lifestyle that contribute to its growth are made available, whenever that may be.

Bo: After my first heart attack in 1969, I was pretty scared. My cardiologist got me to exercise pretty regularly. I started eating better, and I took my medicines real faithfully. But, you know that it's hard to keep that discipline and I was real busy and all. I started back with my bad habits of eating, working all hours, and not getting as much exercise as I should. And you know what? My problem came back.

Jon Falk, Director of Equipment Operations since 1974, described Bo's plan. "Bo studied the heart like it was his football opponent that he was going to be playing against. He studied the doctors, and he knew exactly what was wrong with him, and he knew what had to be done to straighten his challenges out. He knew his weaknesses, and he knew his strengths ...

"He had a challenge and he wanted all the resources he could muster to be ready to win against that challenge."

Symptoms of a Heart Attack

What does a heart attack feel like? Like Bo, most patients describe heart attack pain as a constriction or tightness in the chest. The symptom is frequently located under the breast bone (sternum), but may be perceived on either side of the chest or across the entire chest. The discomfort is most typically described as dull, aching, squeezing, or even like a fullness or bubble. It may also be associated with numbness, tingling, or heaviness in the arms, back, or jaw. Nausea or vomiting occurs in a quarter of patients, shortness of breath in about half, and sweating in a third. The pain may remind the patient of indigestion, a muscle pull, or some prior condition. It may come and go over minutes, only to return minutes or hours later. Women are more likely to experience nausea or vomiting. Many women and some men report profound fatigue in the month before the heart attack.

What Is Heart Disease?

Coronary heart disease is the most common form of heart disease. It occurs when the coronary arteries, which supply blood to the heart muscle, become narrowed due to a buildup of plaque on the arteries' inner walls. Plaque is the accumulation of cholesterol, fat, and other substances on the lining of the coronary arteries. As plaque continues to build up in the arteries, blood flow to the heart may be reduced. Bo's coronary heart disease likely began in a mild form in his teens and twenties.

Coronary heart disease can lead to a heart attack. A heart attack develops if a cholesterol-rich plaque erodes and exposes its contents to the bloodstream. This causes a blood clot to form over the plaque, totally blocking blood flow through the artery and preventing oxygen from getting to the heart. A heart attack can cause permanent damage to the heart muscle. Thankfully, Bo's first heart attack, although dramatic in presentation, left him with only minimal damage to the pumping muscle of his heart.

Besides heart attacks, Bo battled several other types of heart conditions.

Angina

Many Americans live with angina, which is chest pain or discomfort that occurs when the heart muscle is not getting enough blood, a state known as ischemia. Ischemia can be silent or cause symptoms. An episode of angina is not a heart attack, but patients who experience angina are more likely to have a heart attack than those who do not have angina.

One type of angina is called *stable angina.* It may feel like pressure or a squeezing in the chest. The pain may also occur in the shoulders, arms, neck, jaw, or back. Sometimes it feels like indigestion. Other patients experience exertional shortness or tightness of breath as their "angina equivalent." Stable angina is generally brought on by some kind of stress, exertion, or emotion, and it is usually relieved by rest or medicine. Many patients describe a reproducible pattern of angina where, whenever they experience a certain type of stress, their symptoms will recur. Late in his life, Bo was bothered by mild exertional chest tightness when working out or during other activities. This was stable angina. On occasion, when it didn't stop right away, he would take a nitroglycerin tablet to relieve it. Angina can be annoying, but it's the body's signal to stop or slow down and avoid further trouble.

Unstable angina is more serious than stable angina. This may start at any time and often reflects a change in a patient who previously had stable angina. Episodes of unstable angina tend to be more frequent, painful, and persistent than those of stable angina and are less often relieved by rest or medications. Unstable angina is a condition that may evolve into a heart attack. The symptoms are the same as if having a heart attack. Bo's initial symptoms at the 1970 Rose Bowl began as unstable angina. First, he noted chest pressure running drills with the team. Then, his chest pressure sensation would not go away and, when severe, stopped him from walking up a hill. Finally, he had persistent chest pressure and indigestion, indicating his heart attack.

Tests to Identify Coronary Artery Disease

The one thing we can all count on is that the longer we live the better the technology will become to help diagnose and treat cardiovascular disease. Bo benefited greatly by the technological advances that were made in his lifetime. That said, we do not always get the proper diagnoses, even when the human element is removed from the decision making. Continued advances in technology are improving the diagnosis of cardiac incidents, as well as the treatment of cardiovascular disease.

Bo: I was so surprised in 1969 to learn that an EKG can be inaccurate immediately after a heart attack. Why is that? You would think it would show up immediately.

Bo's initial heart attack in 1969 was a small one, and it did not show up on his initial electrocardiogram. We now know that the heart doesn't always show the changes after a heart attack, and some heart attacks never show up on an EKG at all. If the heart damage is in the back of the heart, and we are taking EKGs that mainly identify problems in the front of the heart, it is electrically "silent," and the EKG may not show it. So sometimes we need to use blood enzyme or cardiac marker tests to diagnose a heart attack.

The blood markers become elevated when heart muscle cells are damaged. If a patient was having bad angina spells that went away on their own and didn't have an EKG during an episode when the patient was having the angina discomfort, then the patient might get falsely reassured that nothing bad had happened. This happened to Bo the day before his heart attack was diagnosed. An EKG taken *during* symptoms often allows the doctor to see evidence that the heart muscle is feeling starved for oxygen, but even then, sometimes, the EKG looks fine.

Many people think they might have heart disease but they're not sure. As happened to Bo, heart disease doesn't always announce itself with symptoms. His coronary artery blockages were severe and multiple before he even became aware that there was a problem. That means a person could have heart disease and still feel perfectly fine. A patient should consult with their doctor about their personal degree of heart disease risk and about whether getting tested to look for "silent" coronary heart disease is a good idea.

Most screening tests for heart disease are done outside of the body and are painless. After taking a careful medical history and doing a physical examination, the doctor may order one or more of several tests.

An **electrocardiogram** (ECG or EKG) makes a graph of the heart's electrical activity as it beats. This test can show abnormal heart beats, patterns suggestive of heart muscle damage or poor blood flow, and heart chamber enlargement. However, the ECG will usually not show any problem in patients with intermittent angina, unless the test is performed during an episode. This is what occurred with Bo the day before the 1970 Rose Bowl. When his ECG was obtained, his chest pressure had gone away, so the ECG results were normal.

A **stress test** (or treadmill test or exercise ECG) records the heart's electrical activity during exercise, usually during exercise on a treadmill or exercise bike. For a patient unable to exercise due to arthritis or other health conditions, there are several types of stress tests that can be done without exercise. Instead, a medicine can be given that increases blood flow to the heart muscle that, when combined with specialized imaging of the heart, can show whether any coronary artery blockages are likely to be present.

A **nuclear heart scan** (thallium or sestamibi stress test) shows the status of the heart muscle as blood flows through the heart. A small amount of radioactive material is injected into a vein, usually in the arm, and a specialized camera records how much of the radioisotope enters the heart muscle. Areas of reduced uptake suggest that there may be a narrowing in the coronary artery supplying that region of the heart.

Echocardiography (echo stress test) is a technique in which sound waves are directed at the heart and then analyzed to create a two-dimensional picture of the heart's size, shape, and motion. When combined with a treadmill exercise test, or after intravenous infusion of a medication that mimics exercise, an echo stress test helps identify severe blockages in the coronary arteries, areas of heart muscle damage, and narrowing as well as leaking of the heart valves.

Coronary angiography (angiogram or arteriography) shows a movie X-ray of blood flow in the coronary arteries and identifies any major blockages. A thin, flexible tube called a catheter is threaded through an artery of an arm or leg up into the heart. A dye is then injected through the catheter, allowing the heart and blood vessels to be filmed as the heart pumps. The picture is called an angiogram or arteriogram. Because this type of test involves threading a catheter into a major artery and into the heart's coronary arteries, it is considered to be an invasive test and carries with it a small risk of causing a heart attack, stroke, and, in very rare cases, death.

Carotid Doppler ultrasound uses sound waves to detect narrowing of the carotid arteries in the neck. Patients with cholesterol plaques in the carotid arteries may also have coronary artery blockages. Similarly, patients with cholesterol blockages in the heart's coronary arteries may develop blockages in the carotid arteries that can predispose patients to the risk of stroke. Bo had moderate blockages in both his carotid arteries, but thankfully, he never suffered a stroke. His degree of carotid artery blockage was monitored annually with Doppler ultrasound studies.

Computed tomography (CT) is a superfast scan that provides a three-dimensional picture of the coronary arteries. The first type of cardiac CT scan used a technique called electron beam imaging (EBCT) to determine whether there was a calcium buildup in the walls of the coronary arteries. It provides a coronary calcium score: the higher the score the higher the risk for a heart attack. The latest technique is a 64-slice CT scan of the heart that allows doctors to not only detect areas of calcium buildup in the coronary arteries but also non-calcified plaque buildup. This offers the possibility of getting a coronary angiogram without having to use an invasive catheter to inject the dye into the heart's coronary arteries. Coronary calcium scores and/or 64-slice CT coronary angiography can be used to help in deciding who to treat with cholesterol-lowering drugs. The CT angiogram is not generally done as a routine screening test because of the radiation exposure, but can be very helpful in persons with symptoms. This may change as the technology improves, the price becomes more affordable, and insurance providers change their coverage of cardiac screening tests.

Magnetic resonance imaging (MRI) of the heart also offers future promise as a noninvasive method to examine the coronary arteries. Currently, it is mostly used to look for inherited diseases of the heart muscle, tumors, and problems with the lining around the heart (the pericardium).

Recovering from My First Heart Attack— Recruiting from My Living Room!

We have learned a great deal about the causes and treatments of heart attacks since Bo's first heart attack in 1969. Like so many "injuries" to the body, the medical community was conservative on mobility for most any heart injury. That certainly was the case for Bo when he returned home in January of 1970. Today, the medical community sees the benefits of improved circulation for the healing process once the injury has stabilized.

Rudy Reichert, Bo's former cardiologist, remembers, "After Bo got home from California in January 1970, I went over to his house. He was looking me over, I was looking him over, and Millie was looking us both over! He said, 'I want to go back to work. I want a doctor that will get me back to coaching. Can you do that?' I said, 'All doctors want to get their patients back to work, if they want to go back to work, so I expect to get you back to work.' He said, 'Okay, you're hired.' "

Bo: I give my doctors all the credit for giving me a chance to have a good full life. They never indicated that I would not coach again. After that heart attack, I went into strict training. I walked or ran most days. I ate better, and I lost 22 pounds!

Lynn Koch, Bo's assistant at the time, describes his return to the office: "Bo was home for about two or three months, and then he came into work, and you could tell he had a little bit of a change. He would eat a little bit better; he paced himself a little better as far as not staying quite as late at night. But then the next year, recruiting started again, and he reverted to his old workaholic behaviors."

Bo: After getting back to Ann Arbor, they told me not to do a lot of traveling. So, I recruited out of my living room at home! It's funny. Woody stayed in touch throughout the recruiting season and would stop in to see me, as did my good friend Alex Agase [former head coach at

Purdue and Northwestern and volunteer coach for Bo].
Alex stopped in to see me and to tell me I'm the only head
coach not out on the road. And I told him, "Hey, this is a
good deal man; I've got a real legitimate excuse."

Spring practice that March of 1970 found Bo using a
golf cart to get around and watch practice from the sideline. Nonetheless, Bo's stamina got tested. Quarterback
Jim Betts was throwing the ball to a wide receiver in a
defensive back drill designed to teach the players how to
intercept the ball. Jim threw the ball a little too far, and
Bo, who was sitting in a chair, got run over by defensive
back Tom Darden! Bo is on the ground and all the players fear that he has been killed by the impact. The team
runs over to see how Bo is. Bo is lying on the ground with
eyes closed. Then he starts to move, opens his eyes, and
says, "That would have killed an ordinary man!" This is a
statement his teams heard many times through the years
to show his toughness.

Tirrel Burton, former assistant coach, noticed changes
after Bo's return. "Eventually Bo slowed down on his crazy
schedule, and he became more diet conscious. We used to
work until 11:30, 12 o'clock at night, and be back at 7 or
8 o'clock the next day. Eventually Bo said, 'We are going
home at 10:30.' And you know, you'd really be getting after
it, and some of the guys didn't want to leave, but he would
say, 'Okay, it's 10:30, we're going home.' And he'd get up,
turn out the light, and go home. He became more meticu-
lous about what he ate, too."

Heart Healthy Diets

There are not many of us who enjoy eating a good meal
more than Bo did! As disciplined as he was, it was a tremen-

dous fight to push good food away, especially at the end of a long day or when he felt he had earned a good meal. Like so many of us, Bo knew what he should and should not eat, and most of the time he was pretty good. But then, there were the times when he could not resist. Perhaps that is what helped motivate him to push himself for an hour everyday on the treadmill, bike, or NuStep. Good food was difficult for Bo to push aside, but for the most part his wife Cathy did not let food take control as it may have had she not been monitoring Bo's diet.

One of those times he did not resist was on a recruiting trip with Tirrel Burton. "He told me once he was going to fire me. We went up to Flint to see a recruit and his mom, and we are driving back, and Bo said, 'Tirrel, how long have you been working with me?' I said, 'I don't know, Bo, it's been four or five years.' 'You like your job?' I said, 'Yeah.' He says, 'You see the golden arch up there? If you pass one more McDonalds, you're fired.' He goes in, and he says, 'I'll take a small hamburger, dear, with nothing on it.' Of course, everybody in McDonalds found out who he was, and the waitress came over. 'Would you sign my napkin?' 'Yes, dear, I'll sign that.' He signed that, he looks over at me and says, 'What is that?' I said, 'This is an apple pie for dessert.' He is already eating my French fries, and he says, 'Move that apple pie over a little closer!'"

Bo: Right after the first heart attack I did not let my weight get out of control. It has been up and down. I must say I have always felt better and had more energy when my weight was down, but it is a fight I've had my whole life. My wife Millie was a nurse, and my cardiologist helped us by telling us what I should be eating, but we know a lot more today than we did in 1970.

Prior to his first heart attack, Lynn Koch remembers that Bo "used to eat all fast foods on recruiting trips. He just kept eating, and he didn't exercise a whole lot. He learned that he had to change those habits. If you look at pictures from back in 1969, he looked much better later in life than he did then."

Achieving a heart healthy diet in a culture dominated by fast foods, quick fixes, and the latest diet pill is no easy task. Bo, like many of us, struggled to both maintain his weight *and* a healthy diet for nearly four decades. He discovered that winning with his diet is just like winning at football: you need to work every day to win on Saturday.

Pritikin, Ornish, South Beach, Atkins—these are all famous diet plans that, by and large, work for some people but, overall, skirt the most fundamental problem with America's diet. We eat too much food! And, we don't exercise enough! Study after study has shown that the first and most fundamental issue is how many calories are consumed in a day or a week and how many we expend. Fundamentally, this is the reason why rigorous compliance with a program like Weight Watchers is successful. By counting points, or calories, a person is able to create a situation where calories expended exceed calories consumed, resulting in weight loss. The obesity epidemic in the United States has less to do with what we eat and more to do with how much we eat and how fast. So the first goal of a heart healthy diet is aimed at achieving a daily caloric intake that allows us to maintain a reasonable body weight.

The story of how fast we eat plays into this theme. Each of us has a neurologic connection between our stomach and the satiety center in our brain. When you fill your stomach with food, a message that says "You're full" is received by the brain, telling you to stop eating. But there's a problem. On average, it takes 15 to 30 minutes for your brain to get this message! So, if we eat quickly, most of us eat more than we would if we ate slowly and, as a result, we gain weight. We eat in a manner that rarely gives this natural internal feedback loop a chance to tell us that we were full 10 minutes ago!

Of course, quality of food is important for heart patients like Bo Schembechler. His diet was dually complicated by a need to try to control blood sugar and lower his LDL or bad cholesterol. It starts by eating foods that are low in fat, especially saturated and trans-fats, which are especially harmful to coronary patients. Eating a nice, consistent balance of fruits, vegetables, whole grains, and poultry and fish becomes very important. Having more, not less, fiber is also helpful. Cholesterol content is generally less important than fat content. Refer to the American Heart Association's web site for additional information on diet and nutrition, www.americanheart.org. Marketing strategists try to trick us when they advertise "no cholesterol" potato chips, for example, when they fully understand that high-fat potato chips are generally less healthy than high-cholesterol eggs!

Current Heart Healthy Diet Recommendations
Nutrient Targets for Patients with Coronary Heart Disease

Nutrient	Recommended Intake
Total calories (energy)	Balance energy intake and expenditure to maintain desirable body weight
Saturated fat plus trans-fatty acids	Less than 7% of total calories
Polyunsaturated fat	Up to 10% of total calories
Monounsaturated fat	Up to 20% of total calories
Total fat	25–35% of total calories
Carbohydrates	50–60% of total calories
Fiber	20–30 grams per day
Protein	Approximately 15% of total calories
Cholesterol	Less than 200 milligrams per day

In addition to eating the right foods and the right quantity, Bo learned "when" he ate was also important. By eating a healthy breakfast followed by smaller, healthy meals spaced evenly throughout the day, his blood sugar, triglyceride, and cholesterol levels were more consistent. This eating pattern increases stability of calorie consumption and expenditure from day to day. This helped to reduce Bo's weight variation, helped his blood sugar stay consistent, and reduced the progression of coronary heart disease.

Heart Healthy Physical Activity

We hear from those who do not like to exercise that their hearts only have so many beats in them, and they are preserving their beats by not working out. Well ... research has shown that that is not the case. Bo's cardiologist Dr. Rudy Reichert states he knew 40 years ago that those who kept their heart active had fewer cardiovascular disease issues, long before research supported his hypothesis.

Dr. Reichert feels that "Bo was a wonderful example of hope for others on how statistics do not always apply." He explains that "Bo had these terrible arteries and other cardiovascular problems, and statistics say he should have died early from his disease. He'd worn out two exercise bicycles, never smoked, and never abused alcohol. A human is like a frog, most of his muscle is in his legs. If you convince yourself that you like walking and do it, you will get real cardiovascular benefits. You do not need to do marathons to get cardiovascular benefits."

Mary Passink remembers Bo "jogging for an hour on the treadmill, until later in his life when his diabetic neuropathy got so bad. He had a little TV, mounted above his treadmill, and he'd watch CNN, the stock market, and other news. Then he went to the bicycle due to his neuropathy. When they went to Florida, he worked out at the club in the morning doing his jogging and lifting weights. Then he would eat lunch, and he would go back and do a little bit more. He had this drive to heal himself. Cathy was worried he might kill himself working out. But in the back of his mind he thought that 'If I do this, it's going to give me a little bit more time to live.' He was so determined."

According to Jerry Hanlon, a former assistant coach, "Bo was one of the most disciplined persons that you were ever going to be around, not only with people he dealt with, but with himself. That's one of the attributes that he had—if he knew he had to work out, somehow he was going to find time to work out. That discipline he demanded of others he also demanded of himself. He was ornery enough that he wanted to stay around and enjoy life as long as he could because he worked awful hard to get where he was."

Dr. Reichert attributes Bo's diet and exercise with adding years to his life. "The lack of toxins in his diet and his faithful exercise reduced his stress and stimulated collateral growth of his coronary arteries. Blood vessels do not grow unless you create a need, and then the little capillaries can turn into larger arteries, but they won't do that unless you create a need. That's one thing that Bo had been very faithful about after he retired. In a way, by maintaining a significant and dedicated exercise routine, he created his own bypass grafts where the ones we placed surgically failed.

"If you like your job, you want to go back to work, like Bo did, and that motivated him to coach himself back to health. Bo would tell me, 'Doc, I ride that bike all the time, I'm exercising, and before I came up here, I rode for an hour.' He rode a bike longer than most people. He was such a competitor. If he had to do a stress test he would ask,

'What have the previous guys done? What's good?' Then he would do one better. And it hurt to do it, and then upon returning he would ask, 'What was it before, because I have to beat that.' He was always a competitor.

"The unique thing about his exercise was that he would exercise until he had angina. Then, with a little patience, it would ease off and he'd keep going. Studies now show that exercise up to a certain point, where the heart is beginning to feel a limitation in blood flow, is actually a strong stimulation to form new coronary artery branches in at-risk zones (oxygen-deprived areas of the heart). Bo never gave up. He kept working out every day and kept looking for solutions. Even when he had bad days and was discouraged, he never, ever gave up."

To protect our hearts, we must keep moving. For people with heart disease, physical activity greatly decreases the risk of the disease getting worse. Lack of physical activity can also worsen other heart disease risk factors, such as high blood pressure, diabetes, and being overweight.

Studies show that as little as 30 minutes of moderate-intensity physical activity three or four days a week helps to protect heart health. This level of activity can reduce the risk of heart disease complications and lessen the risk of having a stroke, high blood pressure, and difficult-to-control diabetes. For exercise to also assist in weight loss, longer and more intense workouts (e.g., 45 to 60 minutes) are more effective.

Examples of moderate exercise include taking a brisk walk, light weightlifting, dancing, raking leaves, washing a car, housecleaning, riding a stationary bike or rowing machine, or gardening. If one prefers, it's fine to divide the 30-minute activity into shorter periods of at least 10 minutes each. Some people who walk for their exercise like to use a pedometer to log daily activity rather than measuring time. Ten thousand steps a day roughly translates into a 30-minute sustained walk at moderate pace, plus daily activity. Thus, either 30 minutes a day or 10,000 steps a day are the minimum goals for heart disease prevention.

Faith

Faith played a major role in Bo's life. As a young boy, he was the acolyte of his Episcopal Church in Barberton, Ohio. The commitment to his church continued in Ann Arbor, and wherever he was, he felt he should be doing more as a Christian.

Bo: I was the acolyte anytime I was in town. If I came home from college, I was the acolyte. It meant a great deal to me to be a part of that church.

But Bo had high expectations of everyone, especially himself.

Bo: I've been a slacker when it comes to being the Christian I desire to be. I grew up Episcopalian. There was one acolyte that ran the show in our little Episcopal Church in Barberton, Ohio ... Me. The only time that I wasn't there was when I was away at college. If I came home on vacation, I'm there. After I left there, I never really got involved in a church the same way, and I don't know why.

But those who attended 8 o'clock Communion services at St. Andrew's Episcopal Church in Ann Arbor could see Millie doing the first reading, and Bo doing the second reading, and Shemy serving as the acolyte.

Bo's abiding belief that his "mission" was to serve his family, players, friends, and the university was a strong, deeply held belief that expressed itself throughout his life.

The Second Quarter—1976–1989

Return of Heart Symptoms

The scare of the heart attack the day before the 1970 Rose Bowl had worn off, and Bo had returned to a pace of life his heart could not support. Like his preparation for a formidable opponent, Bo did his research to understand what he was up against and developed the best game plan available for the proper attack. There were no stones left unturned by Bo to find the best answers and ensure the best results possible.

Bo: I felt some chest tightness in the spring of 1976. So they catheterized me, studied the results, and then all of the docs gathered around and said, "We think we ought to operate." And I said, "Well, what do you do when you operate?" They said, "Well, you ought to talk to the guy we recommend, Dr. Otto Gago." So Otto comes in and he takes the angiogram film and goes through it with me and shows how he is going to put four or five bypasses in. "We will put one there," and then he showed me what he is going to do. Then I said, "You know, in my business it's best if you get some additional advice on big decisions and some other opinions about whether this is the right thing to do or not." I took the films with me, and I went to Cleveland, to a doctor recommended by my good friend Joe Hayden in Cincinnati, and to Houston.

You don't just say, "Boy this looks like the thing to do, just go ahead and do it." You get a lot of expert advice. It's like in football, if it's a radical change in offense and defense, you are going to do it in the off season, and you are going to go talk to some of the top guys around that you are not competing against, saying, "Take a look at this. I got this idea. What do you think?" So, I felt by the time I got ready for the operation, I had done my homework. I knew where I was and where I was going.

Rudy Reichert remembers Bo's travels for other opinions: "After his angiogram, the first thing he did, he got a suitcase, and he took his catheterization data, and he connected with all those friends in high places on what he should do. Like everything he did, he thought hard about his options and he talked to everybody. He talked to Denton Cooley, he went everywhere. He told me, 'I knew I was coming back here, but I just wanted to feel comfortable about it.' He's a smart guy. He wasn't going to just take the first recommendation. So he gave the decision a lot of scrutiny, then he came back and, luckily, residing in Ann Arbor was a surgical genius by the name of Otto Gago. Surgeons tell me that it was a symphony watching him operate. He was so skilled, and all of his peers said the same thing.

Tirrel Burton also recalls Bo's journey. "Bo dove into health care just like he did football. When he first was having his problems, he'd go out and get every book he could find, and he would read and learn about it. Before his first operation, he asked Dr. Gago, 'Now, I've been reading about this. What do you think, and how are you going to do this operation?' The doctor replied, 'You get to bed the night before, and be ready for a big game.' Dr. Gago is Venezuelan and speaks with a very strong accent. And he goes to assure Bo he is up for the challenge, and says, 'Don't worry, Bo, it's a cup of cake.' And Bo responds, 'It's not a cup of cake … it's a *piece* of cake!' "

Procedures for Managing
Coronary Heart Disease

Advanced coronary heart disease can often be mitigated by special procedures to open or bypass a blocked artery and improve blood flow to the heart muscle. As in Bo's case, these operations are usually done to ease severe chest pain or reduce coronary artery blockages. Examples of commonly performed cardiac procedures include coronary angioplasty, stent placement, and coronary bypass surgery.

Coronary Angioplasty or "Balloon" Angioplasty

In this procedure, a thin tube called a catheter is threaded through an artery into the narrowed heart vessel. The catheter has a tiny balloon at its tip, which is inflated to open and stretch the artery. Then the balloon is deflated and the catheter removed. This process improves blood flow to the heart muscle beyond the blockage, thus reducing chest pain and helping to prevent a heart attack.

Compared with coronary bypass surgery, the advantages of angioplasty are that the procedure is less invasive, the patient receives local anesthesia only, and the recovery period is shorter. The disadvantage is that, in some cases, the artery narrowing recurs shortly after the procedure. The other issue is that the procedure only treats one segment of a coronary artery that in fact may have mild or moderate atherosclerotic plaque throughout the entire artery.

In many cases, coronary angioplasty is a planned procedure. But it is also used as an emergency treatment during a heart attack to open a blocked coronary artery quickly. If performed early after a heart attack begins, the procedure restores blood flow and minimizes injury to the jeopardized heart muscle.

Stent Placement

A stent is a tiny wire mesh tube (like mini-chicken wire!) that is used to prop open a formerly narrowed artery. A stent is commonly used along with balloon angioplasty. In this procedure, a stent is slid over a balloon catheter and then moved into the area of the blockage. When the balloon is inflated, the stent expands into place, holding open the artery. The stent remains in the artery permanently and reduces the chance that the artery will renarrow.

Currently, most implanted stents are coated with a medication that is slowly released and helps to keep the blood vessel from closing up again. Medications are usually taken to prevent blood clotting on the stent. After implantation of a drug-eluting stent, patients are encouraged to take both aspirin and another anticlotting medication, clopidogrel, for at least a year to reduce the chance of clotting of this type of stent. Current drug-eluting stents reduce early artery renarrowing as compared to bare-metal stents. However, this early benefit may be somewhat offset by a late risk of the stent clotting unless both aspirin and clopidogrel are maintained long term.

Coronary Bypass Surgery

Bypass surgery is often used when coronary artery blockages are too numerous or extensive to allow for coronary stenting or are too firm or hazardous for stenting to be effective. In bypass surgery, the surgeon typically uses pieces of veins from the leg to replace the diseased coronary artery. In some patients, one or both mammary arteries lining the inside of the chest wall are sewn to the heart arteries below the areas of narrowing. Both procedures create a path for blood flow around the blockage. In recent years, with coronary stenting becoming more effective and safe, coronary bypass surgery is reserved primarily for situations where all three major coronary artery territories have a major blockage, or when the location or shape of the narrowing makes angioplasty with stenting impossible or too risky.

Although vein grafts are very effective bypass choices for the short term, they may become blocked from cholesterol and scar buildup over a decade or so. Internal mammary artery bypass grafts are usually more durable, often working well for a couple of decades. In Bo's case, his first bypass procedure involved the use of multiple vein grafts harvested from his leg. Studies of bypass graft durability had not yet shown that using the mammary arteries was any better than using veins. Just eleven years later, all his original vein grafts were blocked! His second bypass included placement of two mammary artery bypass grafts, as well as more vein grafts. Nineteen years later, one of the two mammary artery grafts was still open, representing the major blood supply to Bo's heart. All his vein grafts and the other mammary artery graft were closed.

Bo: Bypass surgery was like being run over by a truck. It hurt! Then you have the stitches on your legs from where they took the vein grafts and in your chest where they got to your heart, and tubes into you. After the first surgery, I no sooner woke up than I saw Les Miles (who went on to be head coach at Oklahoma State and Louisiana State University) was looking down at me! I don't know how

*he got through everybody. He was looking down at me,
and I thought "I hope I have not upset Lester recently,"
as he had a pretty good temper!*

Recovery after a Heart Attack or
Heart Revascularization
(Angioplasty or Bypass Operation)

It takes time to recover after a heart attack or a heart revascularization. When Bo had his first heart attack in early 1970, and his bypass operation in 1976, he was "grounded" at home for six weeks after the events! Nowadays, patients are mobilized much more quickly, often discharged in just 3 or 4 days, walking up to a mile within a week or two, and enrolled in cardiac rehabilitation (rehab) programs within a few weeks. The speed of returning to normal activity and exercise depends on the magnitude of heart damage, age of the patient, speed of wound healing, and presence of other illnesses. Physically and emotionally, having a heart attack or heart procedure is a big deal. But the quicker a patient can get back to their normal routine the better.

There are several keys to a rapid and safe recovery. First, the patient needs enough time and space to recover. This means getting enough rest, scheduling time away from usual activities and work, learning how and when to take the heart medications, and adopting more healthy lifestyles. This includes eating a heart protective diet, exercising regularly, avoiding tobacco, and learning what one can and can't do. Bo was always forthright in asking specific questions about all of these aspects of recovery.

Bo: Tell me again about the optimal diet? How much exercise? When can I go back to the office? What about having sex, lifting weights, travel, etc? What do I need to track? What about blood pressure, pulse, blood sugar, weight, and follow-up doctor visits?

By writing the answers to these questions down, and by involving his wife in all of these areas, this reinforced his confidence in how to live and what to watch for in future times.

Today, most patients undergo cardiac rehab to help them recover from a heart attack or heart surgery. Rehab programs for heart health include exercise training, education on heart healthy living, counseling to reduce stress, identification and treatment of depression, further education on the use of proper cardiac medications, and planning a return to a normal life. Cardiac rehab helps to renew a person's confidence in their health, strengthen the heart, reduce the risks of a future heart attack, and improve understanding of each aspect of long-term preventive treatment.

Getting Back to Coaching

After Bo's 1976 bypass surgery, he naturally wondered whether he would be able to return to coaching. Like most people, he was able to return safely to most of his normal activities within a few weeks. He was cautioned to watch for recurrent symptoms like chest pain, shortness of breath, or unusual leg swelling. After his 1969 heart attack, he'd been asked to delegate some of the main coaching duties to his assistant coaches for a while to make sure he would find time for rest, cardiac rehabilitation, and his follow-up medical visits. His doctors also performed a stress test to make sure his heart was functioning at a high level after his 12 weeks of cardiac rehabilitation, and before he really went back to work full-time.

Bo, like other patients, was counseled to wait just a few weeks after his bypass surgery before resuming normal sexual activities. He was told "It's best not to do this after a heavy meal or during times of extreme stress."

In recent years, patients who are sexually active must be counseled on the interaction between drugs for angina (nitrates) and medications used to reduce erectile dysfunction (like sildenafil). These drugs, when used within 24 to 48 hours of one another, may cause a serious drop in blood pressure that can become life-threatening.

Return of Symptoms—1987

Bo was a prototypical "Type A" person who was driven to do all he could to succeed in his profession. As the scare of the heart attack in 1969 had faded over time, likewise memory of the bypass surgery in 1976 had faded, and Bo found himself eating too much, not exercising as much as he should, and pushing the envelope on stress tolerance. This episode in 1987 did get his attention, and he pretty much kept a good focus on his heart health after that time.

Bo: I think it was during the Minnesota game in 1987 that I felt it again. I knew something changed in there. I developed that same chest tightness I'd had at the Rose Bowl in 1969. It was in the same place, same type of pressure. I knew exactly what it was. Yeah, as a matter of fact, I'm not so sure how close this was to that game, but it was immediately following that season, I believe, that they decided to give me a thallium stress test. I said, "Fine." They got me in there, it was late in the afternoon, and so I did the test and they said, "Look, you ought to stay overnight and have Millie come pick you up in the morning." I said, "Okay." So, I'm lying in the bed, reading the paper the next morning and Millie comes in and sits in the chair, and we are waiting for the doctors to release us to go home. And it hit me, and I told Millie without reservation, I said, "Millie, get the doctors quick, I'm having a heart attack."

She ran out there and next thing I know my cardiologist is back here, and they are slapping the EKG on and doing all those things. And then, it so happens, that apparently my cardiac surgeon had the operating room reserved for that morning, and he had done an operation the night before as an emergency, or something like that. He was there with his group and so they went through all of this stuff with me and then, I'll never forget, I think it was my cardiologist that came over and said, "Look, we can't wait any longer, we've got to operate now." I said, "Oh yeah, look, I don't even want to think about this, sedate me fast." And they did, and they sent me in and I had my second heart operation. That's how I had it—as an emergency.

Rudy Reichert remembers the attack in 1987 as "a real surprise. I don't think it was anything he'd done. He just had more angina ... and I suspect he first noted it when he would ride his bicycle. He noticed a change in his cardiac reserve. That's when we decided to repeat his heart catheterization.

"I know the second bypass surgery was very difficult and chancy, and I think because Bo had a super surgeon that it came off pretty well. But Bo was left with significant heart disease. As I recall, all his vein bypasses were closed. But his mammary arteries were okay. We could use them."

The first time Dr. Kim Eagle saw Bo's coronary angiograms, he "was stunned. The one mammary artery graft was open, but all the main arteries and the other vein bypass grafts were shut. I remember looking at the picture and asking myself, 'How can this heart be working?' "

Dr. Otto Gago, Bo's cardiac surgeon, explains how Bo came to have a mammary artery graft. "We always thought about using the mammary arteries even when I was a resident in training in the early sixties, but in the early days of bypass surgery they were rarely used. You know, we had several patients with very good results after using these vessels. Later, you could actually see the collateral arteries forming. I recall two patients where the implanted mammary practically fed the entire coronary artery system. So we always thought that using the mammaries was a better alternative. We were doing them earlier than most other surgical groups.

Bo: My second bypass was an emergency. I mean I was already in the hospital, and I could tell that I was having a heart attack, so I told them, and they wheeled in the EKG, and this and that, and I'll bet you within an hour of that time, I was in the operating room. And it was just lucky that my surgeon was there, you know with his team, and they just wheeled me in and they said, "Well, we are going to have to go in again."

When Bo's symptoms of angina returned in 1987, a little more than a decade after his first bypass operation, there was little doubt in his mind what was going on. While the symptoms of angina may be difficult for patients to describe, most become immediately aware of its return because it is such a distinctive feeling. Surely, most patients feel both frustrated and alarmed when angina symptoms return, especially if they have been on appropriate heart medications, have achieved their lifestyle goals and have undergone previous successful heart surgery.

In Bo's case, a return of his cardiac symptoms was not difficult to explain. Cardiovascular disease was still present. The first bypass surgery in 1976 was a temporary fix, and while his lifestyle was helping to slow it down, the disease was still there. First, since many vein grafts begin to close in later years, one might have expected that when this happened, his chest discomfort would recur.

Second, the years between 1976 and 1987 predated many breakthroughs in both drug-related preventive therapy and understanding the actual benefits of a healthy lifestyle. Bo's blood cholesterol had not been effectively treated in those early years because our ability to lower the bad LDL cholesterol was not very good—that is, until the first statin, lovastatin, was introduced. His total cholesterol in 1987 was 319 mg/dL, which was very elevated (normal is less than 200 mg/dL).

Third, Bo's diabetes began in the mid-1980s and surely tended to accelerate his coronary artery disease. His fasting blood sugar was 125 mg/dL in 1987 and rose to 172 mg/dL by 1989.

Lastly, although he was taking aspirin and a beta-blocking drug, several newer medications for heart health like the ACE inhibitors, which later helped his heart, kidneys, and arteries, and angiotensin receptor blocking (ARB) agents, which also have multiple benefits for a patient like Bo, were not yet available.

Having a second bypass operation also became a powerful reminder for Bo to achieve maximal lifestyle goals to try to stop his coronary artery disease progression. For Bo, his ability to shut out stress was especially important in his profession.

Bo: When I understood that some of the previous bypasses had closed up, that tells you these are not going to last forever. You have to change something in your lifestyle, or you are not going to make it.

Lloyd Carr noticed a change after the second surgery. "I saw a new discipline in regards to the way he ate. When I first joined Bo's staff, Bo loved to eat. So we would go on the road recruiting and he liked hamburgers and cheeseburgers and pizza. But after the 1987 open heart surgery he changed."

Stress and the Heart

Stress and heart disease are connected in several ways. A common trigger for a heart attack is an emotionally upsetting event. Also, many people respond to stress in harmful ways such as overeating, smoking, or drinking excess alcohol. For people with heart disease, regular physical activity helps to reduce stress and lowers the risk of heart disease complications. Stress management programs also help prevent recurrent heart attacks.

Strong social support is important to improve recovery after a heart attack. Bo was fortunate in that he managed stress in his life with tremendous effectiveness. His brutal honesty kept his conscience clear. He loved what he did, but he left the football games on the field. He napped in his office every day at work. He stayed physically active later in his life. He had an endless network of former players, coaches, and friends to help him stay on track with his health goals and to share his good moments and the more challenging ones. He had very supportive wives, first Millie and then, later in his life, Cathy, who were tremendous advocates for achieving his health goals and for seeking medical care when signs of problems arose.

Dan Ewald, former Detroit Tigers media relations director and coauthor of *Michigan Memories,* believes that "when people are open, like Bo, they save themselves a lot of stress. Bo was in a stressful, stressful occupation and because of the personality and the size of the university he represented, he got more exposure. Bo's life was followed by more people across the country than the average celebrity's. Because of Bo's openness and brutal honesty, I think he relieved a lot of stress."

At first, former player and Bo's Director of Operations Fritz Seyferth wasn't sure if Bo had relaxed. "A year after Bo's first surgery, I was back on campus interviewing Michigan engineers and MBA students and had heard about this new, 'mellower' Bo. So I went to a spring practice, and within 15 minutes he grabbed one of those big offensive linemen and started shaking him. He took his hat and threw it on the ground, and I am thinking, 'Bo hasn't mellowed at all.' And then he walks over to go pick up his hat, he sees me, he gives me a wink, like 'That was pretty good, wasn't it!' I thought to myself, 'This guy knows exactly what he is doing!' "

The Third Quarter—
1989–2003

Leaving Michigan football and Michigan athletics was very, very hard for Bo. He loved the kids and the coaches, but he also knew if he wanted to live to fight another battle, he needed to change his lifestyle. So he did. If leaving Michigan athletics was meant to reduce the stress in Bo's life, the move did not come to fruition right away. Bo's presidency of the Detroit Tigers was meant to be a lighter load for him, easing him into retirement. There was no such thing when Bo saw a Tiger team that reminded him of his 1969 Michigan team—a lot of potential with no disciplined strategic plan to be as good as they could. Battling the "traditional thinking" in baseball to get year-round strength training, quality coaches in the minor league teams, and a new Tiger Stadium, Bo found himself skirmishing at every turn, only to find the team being sold and Bo out of a job weeks before Millie died of adrenal cancer.

Retirement and Bear Bryant

Bo: Millie wanted me to retire in 1989 and I was trying to decide at that time what I should do. I knew being the Head Coach and Athletic Director was wearing on me the way I went at it, but we had things going good in the department and on the team. We had a real good nucleus of players. We had already won two Big Ten champion-ships, back to back. So, I was talking about the possibil-ity of waiting a few more years, and then I get back to the Bear Bryant story that had such an impact on me.

The Bear and I became good friends from All-Star games, so I got to know him pretty well, and then he broke the record as the winningest coach of all time. The Bear was asked to coach the East-West Shrine game in San Francisco and he asked me to help him. And I knew Bear ... so I coached the team and he played golf!

One evening, we get back to the hotel from dinner and the phone rings. "You ready to talk?" And I said, "Yeah, come on down Bear." He comes in, sits down, and he says, "Well Bo, aren't you going to offer me a drink?" So, I got a fifth of bourbon and slapped it down. "What do you want with that?" I said. He says, "I want a little Coke." So I got him a Coke. He took a regular drinking glass, filled it half Coke, half bourbon. We talked a long time about his life and many wonderful stories, and he changes his tone and says, "I want to talk about my problems." I said, "Well, go ahead, what problems do you have?"

He said, "'I don't want to go back to the office. I don't want to talk to another prospect. I don't want to coach anymore." I said, "Well everybody in the United States of America and all those people in Alabama figured after you broke the record that you're not going to coach any-more. You've got a simple solution to that, Coach," and I grabbed the phone off the end table and I put it right down in front of him. I said, "All you need to do is to call your president, and say, I've given it a lot of thought, and I've decided it's time for me to retire."

He got up right then and says, "Damn you, you're going to find out exactly what I'm going through now.

You can't just say you're going to retire. If I retire what happens to those 47 people I hired at the University of Alabama? You know what will happen to them? Half of them will lose their jobs. Damn it I can't quit, I've got to go back there."

And so we finished up the conversation, and he left. Now he went back there that next year, and he had an average team, they played Illinois, in the Liberty Bowl, in Memphis, Tennessee. And a month or two after that, he died. He would not quit because of those 47 people he hired at the University of Alabama. I remember thinking, "I do not want to go out like that."

Gary Moeller and I were talking about my retiring. If I were to leave, I'm going to name him head coach, and so I'm talking to him about that possibility. And Mo says, "Make me offensive coordinator, and let me call the plays." If I had been smart I would have done that, but I could not relinquish the offense. I should have said, "Okay Mo, except on certain instances when I think that I want to do a certain thing, you go ahead and call the plays." That could have made it a little easier for me to coach, if I didn't try to do so much, because I was trying to do three things really: run the athletic department, run the team, and run the offense.

I was thinking, "Maybe I don't want to push it too hard." To coach one more year and beat Woody's win record did not mean anything to me. My health was the reason I left, and I thought I could do something for the Detroit Tigers. Staying would have been easy, as we had a great team. We had three Big Ten Championships in our sights with that team and that was a good bunch of kids. I do think leaving football at that time was the smartest thing I did for my health—though at the time I wished I hadn't done it. I left such great material here, it just galls me that I left the greatest offensive line we ever had. We had championships to win with that team!

Losing Millie was a terrible blow. It was 1991 and we were in Hawaii, really just beginning to be able to take time together, which was never possible at Michigan and one of the reasons to retire. We were going to dinner, and she said to me, "Do you mind if I don't go?" I said, "What's up, you're not feeling good?" She says, "No." So I waited one day and she did not feel any better, so I said, "Pack your bag, we're going home." And I took her back home. It turned out to be cancer of the adrenal glands. Dr. Norman Thompson operated on Millie and told me he could not get it all. I was with the Tigers at that time, and we were having our problems there, and then they fired me the week before Millie died.

Creating a Top Medical Defense

The ability to successfully battle chronic medical conditions like angina, diabetes, and high blood pressure starts with creating a winning medical team and then never straying from the medical game plan. Bo Schembechler embodied both the mind and the discipline needed to make that occur. It takes great discipline to eat right, make sure you are on the right medicines, exercise every day, get your cholesterol low, and keep your blood pressure low. When all these occur, then it's like you're nourishing your heart to build new bypasses. In the areas where the coronary arteries are blocked, their neighbors learn that they have to help out, and they grow new blood vessels. When you grow new blood vessels, you "autobypass" essentially. But it all starts with discipline.

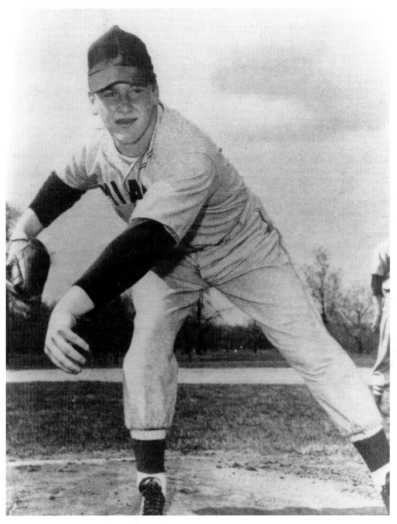

Bo loved baseball, too. By this age, he already very likely had early coronary plaques. (Bentley Historical Library, University of Michigan)

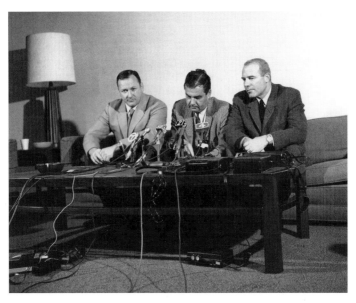

In 1969, Bo Schembechler is named the new Michigan football coach
at a press conference with Don Canham and Bump Elliott.
(Bentley Historical Library, University of Michigan)

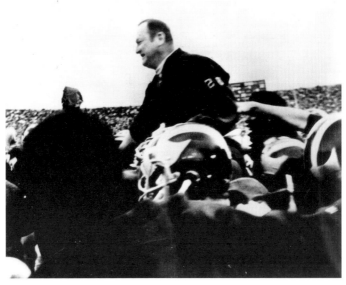

After the 1969 U of Michigan–Ohio State game, Coach Schembechler
was carried off the field by his triumphant team. Within seven weeks
of this day, he would be hospitalized with his first heart attack.
(Bentley Historical Library, University of Michigan)

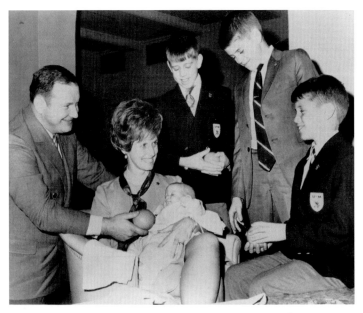

Bo and Millie leaving the hospital with infant Shemy. Chip, Matt, and
Geoff Schembechler welcome their brother with miniature footballs.
(Bentley Historical Library, University of Michigan)

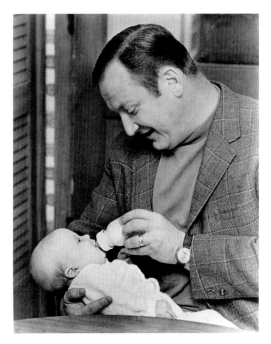

Bo and his son Shemy in 1969
(Bentley Historical Library, University of Michigan)

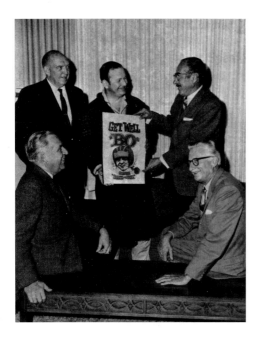

The Tournament of
Roses Committee presents
Bo with get-well wishes at
St. Luke Hospital on
January 16, 1970.
(Bentley Historical Library,
University of Michigan)

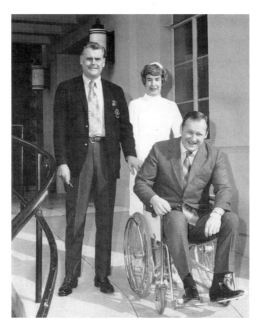

Bo Schembechler leaves St. Luke Hospital in Pasadena, California,
with Hal Coombes (University Entertainment Chairman,
Tournament of Roses) and Mrs. Fowler, R.N., after his first heart
attack before the 1970 Rose Bowl. Remarkably, he would go on to
survive 37 years after that first, potentially fatal, event.
(Bentley Historical Library, University of Michigan)

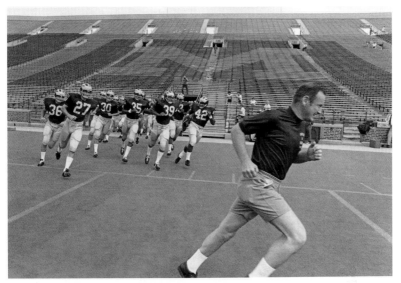

Bo Schembechler leading the U of M team to the field,
Picture Day 1970. A full seven months after his initial heart
attack, Bo is lean and ready for another football season.
(Bentley Historical Library, University of Michigan)

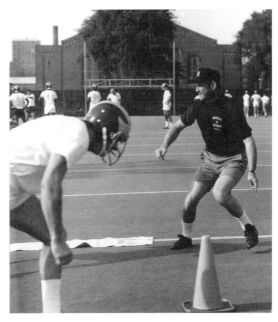

Bo Schembechler at practice in 1970. It was during drills like
this in 1969 that Bo first experienced coronary symptoms.
(Bentley Historical Library, University of Michigan)

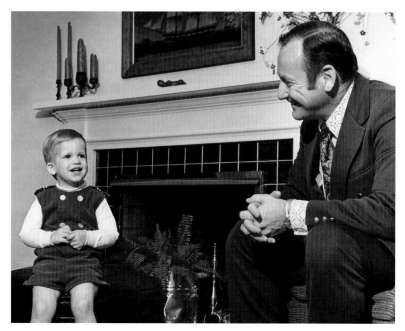

Bo Schembechler with son Shemy, November 20, 1971
(Bentley Historical Library, University of Michigan)

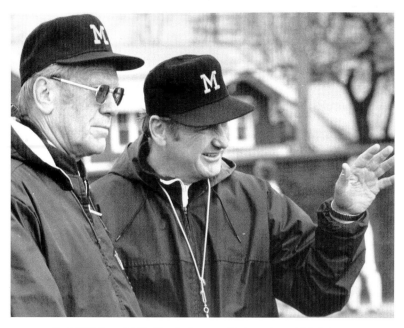

In 1972 Gerald R. Ford, former University of Michigan
captain, visited with Bo at a team practice.
(Bentley Historical Library, University of Michigan)

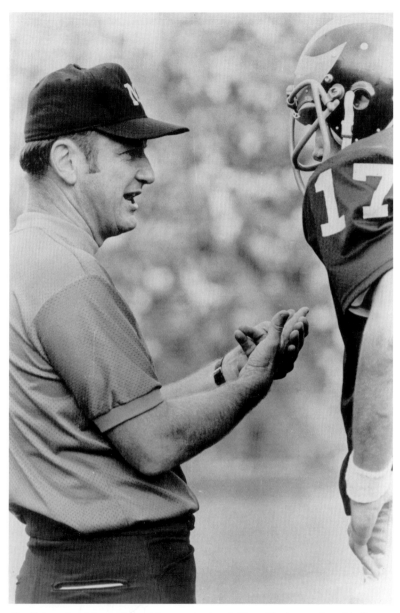

Bo Schembechler talks with quarterback Tom Slade on the sidelines. Bo attended Tom's funeral the day before his own passing in 2006. (Bentley Historical Library, University of Michigan)

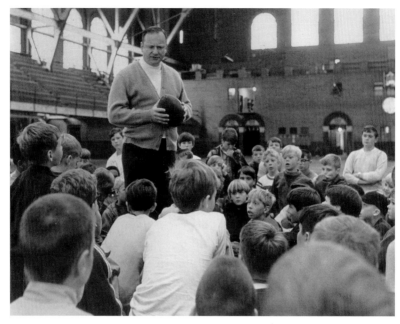

Bo Schembechler speaking to a group of children in 1975.
Bo's love of teaching was an important part of his purpose in life.
(Bentley Historical Library, University of Michigan)

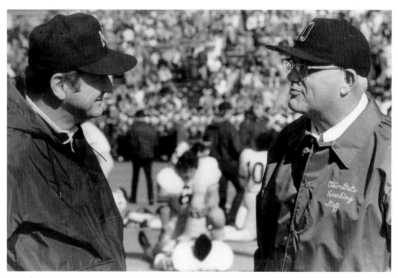

Bo Schembechler and his friend, former mentor, and adversary,
legendary Ohio State coach Woody Hayes in 1976. Like Bo,
Woody fought numerous health battles, including type 2 diabetes.
(Bentley Historical Library, University of Michigan)

Bo, back in full form after his first coronary bypass surgery in 1976, celebrates a 1978 victory over Woody and Ohio State in the Horseshoe in Columbus, Ohio.

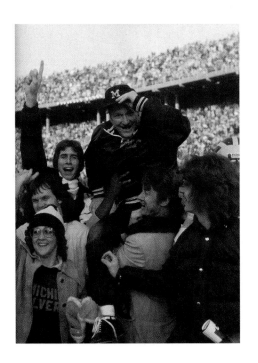

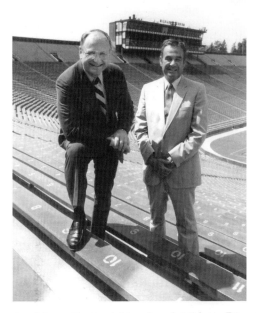

Bo Schembechler with good friend and Athletic Director Don Canham in 1980. The coach is looking lean as he tightened his diet and increased his exercise after his quadruple bypass surgery in 1976. (Bentley Historical Library, University of Michigan)

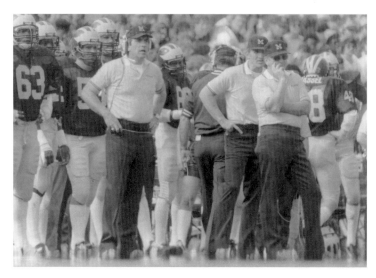

Bo Schembechler with Gary Moeller and Paul Schudel
on the sidelines in 1982 (Bentley Historical Library,
University of Michigan)

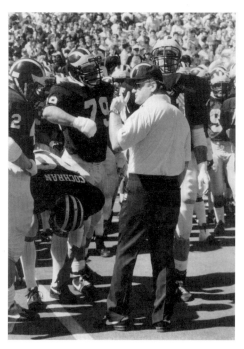

Bo Schembechler was all about building young men through
teaching, by example, and never-ending mentorship.
(Bentley Historical Library, University of Michigan)

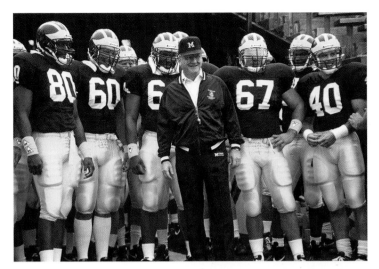

Bo and his team. He developed his medical team with the same discipline and passion. (Photo by Per Kjeldsen)

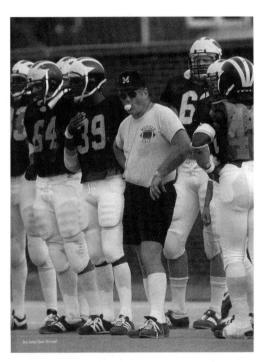

Bo in the 1980s. Maintaining his weight and eating a heart-conscious diet was a challenge during the hectic football season, even after his first bypass surgery. (Tony Tomsic/*Sports Illustrated*)

SPORTS

Bo viewed as invincible

U-M players and coaches and the general public all showed concern for Bo's health during the seven hours of surgery Tuesday, but no one seemed to doubt he'd pull through. More concern was expressed about whether he would coach in the Hall of Fame bowl, how much longer he can coach and whether he'd still be a candidate for athletic director. After all, Schembechler had survived a heart attack and a previous quadruple bypass as if they were nothing more than part of the game plan. Page C1.

In 1987 Bo had been viewed as invincible for as long as we could remember. *(Ann Arbor News)*

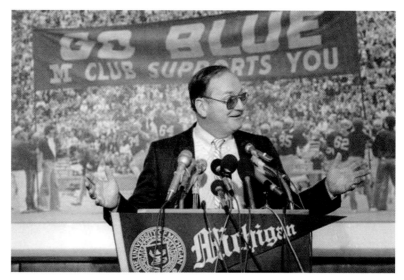

Coach Schembechler announces at a press conference on January 7, 1987, that he intends to continue coaching football after undergoing heart bypass surgery. *(Detroit News/*Donna Terek)

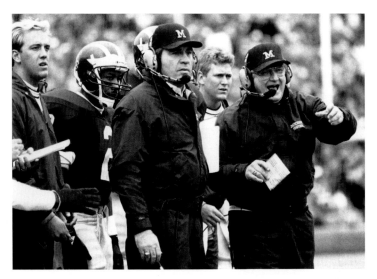

Bo Schembechler and assistant coach Gary Moeller, 1988. That upper body exercise is good for the heart but game-day stress? Probably not! (Bentley Historical Library, University of Michigan)

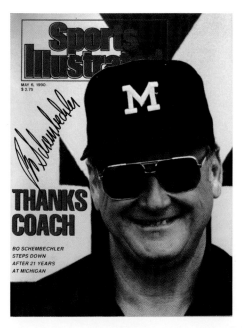

When Bo retired, the University of Michigan hosted a Salute to Bo at Cobo Hall on May 6, 1990, to thank him for his 21 years of service. The back cover of the program was a mock-up of a *Sports Illustrated* cover. (*Sports Illustrated*/Jeanna Cooper Collection)

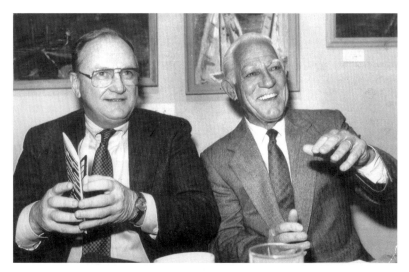

Bo Schembechler and Detroit Tigers manager Sparky Anderson at the Detroit Sports Broadcasters Association meeting at the Detroit Press Club, January 7, 1990. After deciding to step down from the Michigan jobs of Athletic Director and Coach, taking the job of Tigers' president was a tougher challenge than anticipated. (AP/Richard Sheinwald)

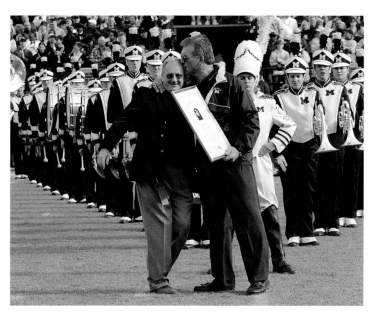

Bo with former player Dan Dierdorf during halftime of a game at the Big House. His former players were always on his mind. (Photo by Per Kjeldsen)

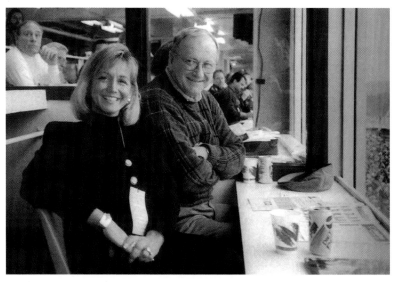

Cathy Schembechler was a huge part of Bo's will to go on.
(Bo Schembechler Collection)

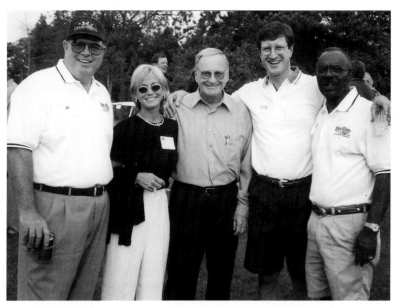

Cathy and Bo Schembechler with *(left)* Jim Brandstatter and
(right) Fritz Seyferth and Tirrel Burton at the thirtieth reunion
of Bo's boys in May 1999. (Courtesy of Jim Brandstatter)

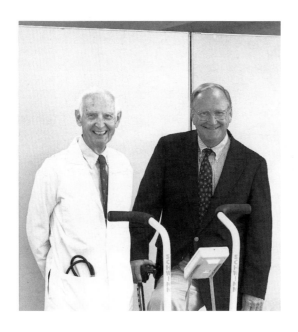

Bo with Rudy
Reichert, his
former
cardiologist

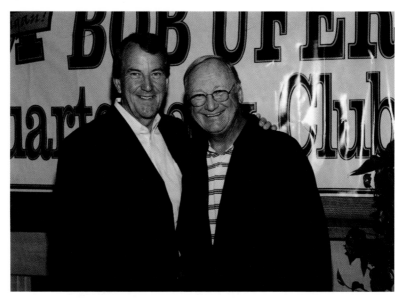

Bo with friend Lloyd Carr. Lifelong friendships were a strong
motivator for his battle to survive. (Photo by Per Kjeldsen)

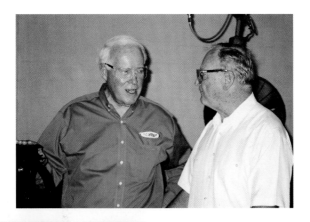

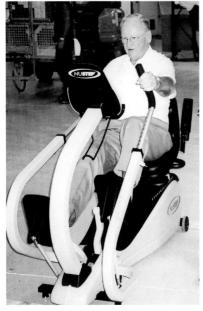

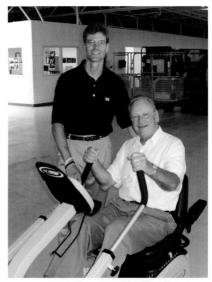

When neuropathy and arthritis made exercising on a treadmill difficult and hazardous, Bo used a NuStep. Dick Sarns, president/CEO *(top),* and Mark Hildebrandt, vice president of research and development *(bottom),* explained the benefits of and how to use the machine. Bo exercised an hour or more each day, right to the end of his life. (Courtesy of NuStep Inc.)

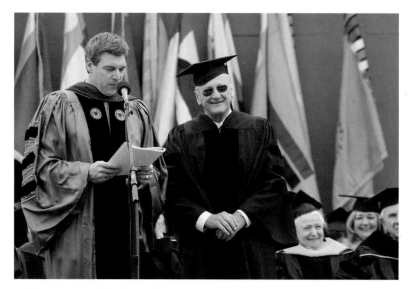

University of Michigan Regent and former University of Michigan football player David Brandon at the 2005 commencement with Bo Schembechler, as Bo receives an honorary degree from the university that became his home and his cause for half of his life. (Photo by Per Kjeldsen)

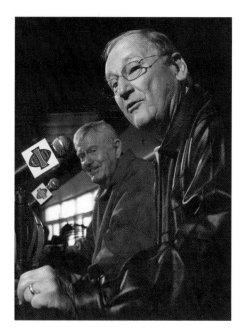

2005 Rose Bowl with legendary Texas coach Darrell Royal. A pacemaker just weeks before gave Bo the boost he needed to get back in the game. (*Detroit News*/Nick Ut)

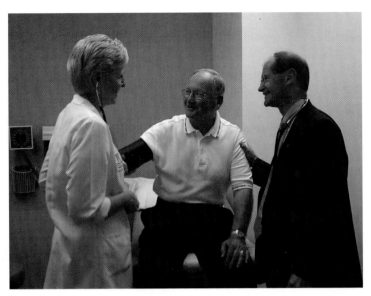

Bo's clinic visits were frequent and focused. He always wanted
to understand each aspect of his case. Nurse Patty Kinaschuk,
Bo Schembechler, and Dr. Eagle, summer 2006.
(U of M Photo Services–Martin Vloet)

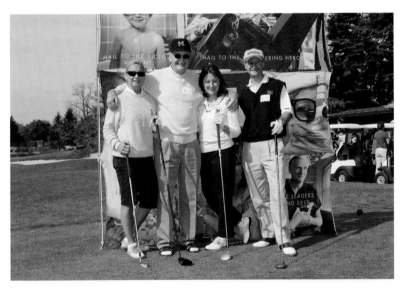

The inaugural Heart of a Champion golf outing occurred on October
9, 2006. Cathy and Bo Schembechler, along with Darlene and Kim
Eagle, are at the first tee. (U of M Photo Services–Martin Vloet)

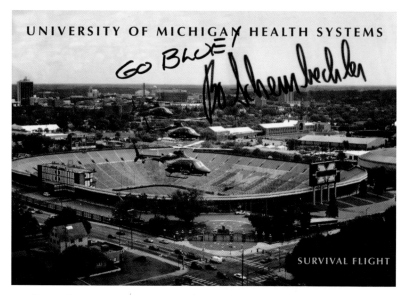

UNIVERSITY OF MICHIGAN HEALTH SYSTEMS

GO BLUE!

SURVIVAL FLIGHT

Bo took a U of M survival flight from an outside hospital to the U of M Medical Center after becoming ill on October 20, 2006. When the nurse asked him how much he weighed, he replied, "Young lady, I'm 195 pounds of blue, twisted steel!" (Courtesy of James Stanley)

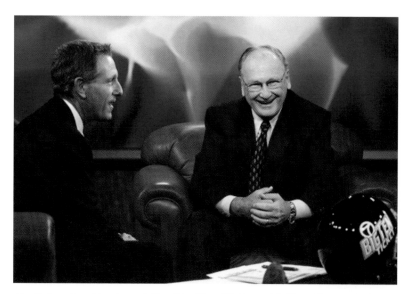

Bo Schembechler taped the *Big Ten Ticket* with Don Shane *(left)* at WXYZ-TV on November 3, 2006. He had been hospitalized October 20 after falling ill at the same location. (*Detroit News*/Charles Tines)

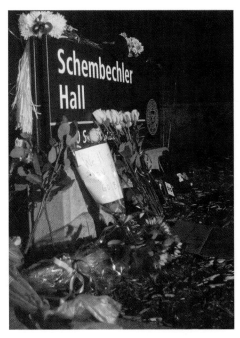

November 22, 2006. A spontaneous informal memorial to Bo
sprang up at Schembechler Hall in the days after his death.
Sixty-three years earlier, at the age of 14, as he watched
Michigan football practice at this very spot, he told his
father that one day he would coach Michigan football.

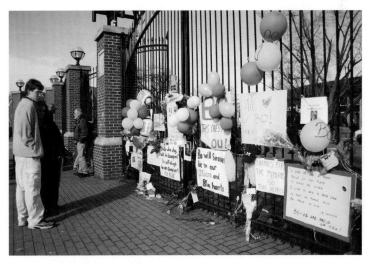

The gates of Michigan Stadium became a shrine in the days
following Bo's death. (Photo by Per Kjeldsen)

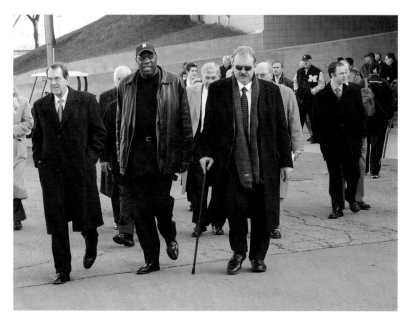

Coach Lloyd Carr and former U of M players Reggie McKenzie and
Dan Dierdorf lead former coaches and players into Michigan
Stadium for a celebration of Bo's life. (Photo by Per Kjeldsen)

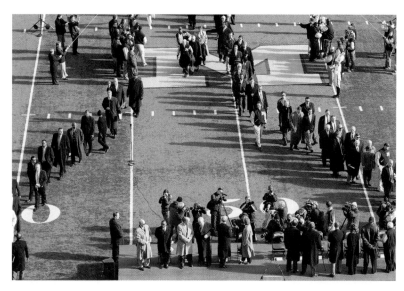

Former players, coaches, and peers by the hundreds converged on
Michigan Stadium for his memorial. (Photo by Per Kjeldsen)

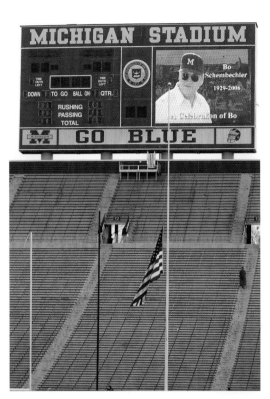

The flag is at half-mast as Michigan mourns for the loss of one of its greats. (Photo by Per Kjeldsen)

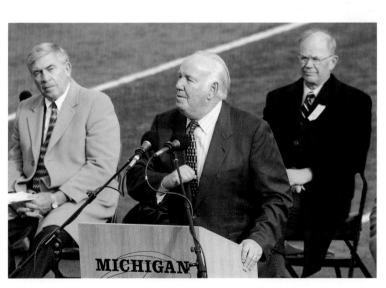

November 21, 2006. Former USC coaching rival and good friend John Robinson remembers Bo with words from the heart. (Photo by Per Kjeldsen)

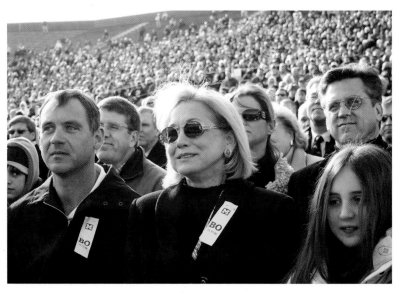

Cathy Schembechler, members of the family, and more than 15,000
people attend Bo's memorial celebration on November 21, 2006,
at Michigan Stadium. (Photo by Per Kjeldsen)

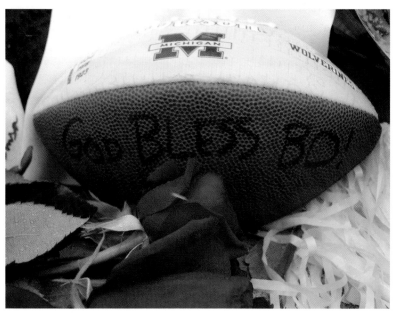

Schembechler Hall, November 19, 2006
(Photo by Jeanna Cooper)

Gary Moeller credits Bo's "success in beating this disease for so long was that he knew how to win. When you know how to win, you know what steps to take, and you don't lose sight of how and why it's important to train. You don't overeat, you have got to walk, and you know it's going to hurt you when you get on that treadmill, but that's how you win. There is sacrifice, too, and he understood sacrifice."

Cathy Schembechler feels "it was Bo's positive attitude and his stubbornness that kept him alive, but most important of all he was disciplined."

Bo on Attitude

Bo epitomized one of his favorite sayings—"What the mind can conceive and believe, the body will achieve." He lived every day with a positive attitude that life just does not get any better, and how lucky we are to be living it. Life was good to Bo, but he made it that way by his passion for living, for touching others' lives, and for making a difference.

Bo: If someone is feeling sorry for themselves, they ought to parade them through a hospital. If you think you have it bad, parade yourself through a hospital. "You are up and walking around for God's sake."

Attitude was always a part of how Bo measured readiness to take on an opponent, and he used it in his fight to stay alive.

Bo: How do people say they have "bad days"? Tell me, how can you have a "bad day"?

Jerry Hanlon, working with Bo as an assistant coach, knew that "Bo's positive attitude in conjunction with his physical conditioning was his strength. Taking ownership of your body is more than thinking about it. You have to push it, you have to sweat it, you have to work it, or you don't get anything."

Alex Agase, former head football coach at Northwestern and Purdue universities and who worked with Bo as a volunteer assistant coach after retirement, remembered Bo's attitude. "Bo was not stubborn, he was just smart. He was told what he had to do, and he did it. He was quite a person. He never acted like he was sick, or depressed, never complained about anything. I didn't even know he had diabetes for a long time. He just didn't complain. He didn't tell you his problems."

Bo's philosophy in dealing with medical challenges was unique. If he was having angina pain half of the time he worked out, he'd think, "Heh, it's only half of the time, which is not bad." Whereas a lot of people, as soon as they start feeling angina, they say, "Oh, it's over. There is nothing I can do."

In the last years of his life Bo said, "I can't say right now that angina was ever a problem. Now, it will come on maybe, but if it does, fine. The truth is that I get a bottle of nitro pills and seldom use them. Now if I was hurting, you know I'd pop one or two in there, you know, to take care of that. But I don't get like that." Bo's angina went away. He built new arteries using the right diet, exercise, and the right medications.

Bo: I believe what they say that if you neglect any one of the three—diet, exercise, and medication—you are not going to make it. One of my favorite sayings is, "What the mind can conceive and believe, the body will achieve." You have got to keep your hopes up. This is medical science, there is always hope around the corner. What you are doing for yourself today, they may have something better tomorrow. It doesn't take long. I've always believed that if you live long enough to keep up with medical discoveries you'll live as long and productive a life as you want to. You can never give up hope and you should do all you can to make the best of the time you have. Sure, your legs may be numb, you may be a diabetic taking four shots a day, you may be taking a dozen pills a day, you may have angina every now and then, and you may feel lousy but the easiest thing to do is to give up. It is easy to say, "What the hell, man ... one thing after another?" How much are you going to tolerate before you say, "It isn't worth it"? That's where you've got to say, "There's no way in hell I won't feel better if I do the right things." Believe it and it is going to happen. It has worked for me!

Rudy Reichert saw the results of Bo's attitude. "Bo had the motivation to get better. He was one of the great motivators of all time. I don't think you can be a motivator unless you can motivate yourself. People catch on to that pretty fast. He defied the statistics. We never had anybody who got along as long and as well as Bo. Nobody. Zero. Bo was unique in the medical practice that I've had in my life. There was no other patient like him."

Jerry Hanlon observes "Bo loved life, and when you look at why he loved life, it's because he was involved in something that he loved to do: helping others, coaching, being around people. And I think that's extremely important if somebody wants to live, it helps to be doing something they like to do. So if you have a heart problem and you hate your job, quit that job and find something you like to do. He just loved his work. He loved to be around kids he could impact.

"Bo had a passion for motivating others to be the best they could be. In his later life he was giving speeches to corporate groups, whether it be the Olympic group in Park City or a high school group, and he still had the ability to motivate and talk straight to any level of people. I know Cathy got mad at him every once in awhile for taking on so many speeches and traveling so much, but he liked helping others.

"His ability to go out and speak gave him purpose in life. He still had his 'game time,' and he enjoyed it. He got to travel; he wasn't sitting home, watching TV, and putting his head down and feeling sorry for himself. Bo was not going to feel sorry for himself. That wasn't going to happen, and that's why he liked those challenges."

Discipline with Medications

Some people fight taking their medications, feeling it is not natural. Bo did not like taking pills either, but he researched each pill and with Cathy's help they read all they could on medications for heart care. He drilled his doctors at each appointment to be sure they knew all the medications he was taking, what this medication would do, and if it would react with other medications he was taking. Bo was disciplined in taking his medications for the most part, but late in life when he did forget to take them on a timely basis, he paid a hefty price. Then Cathy had to play a greater role to be sure Bo took his medications on a timely basis.

Bo: I have had discipline pretty much from the very beginning on taking my medicines. I just figure, I can't fool around with them, and I can't do it in a half-baked way, so I pretty much programmed taking my medications into my life. When you get started you may have one or two pills, and then as you go along, the docs are adding stuff, so you have got to keep up with the regimen of what needs to be taken and when.

My first meds were probably lovastatin for cholesterol and aspirin, but then simvastatin came out right after that. I'm still taking medications for my cholesterol.

Now you talk about discipline, I am disciplined there. I mean, I take those pills the way I'm supposed to take them, and I take them religiously. Now the problem I have is, and I think everybody else with diabetes has it, you take your test and your shot in the morning. Then as afternoon comes and goes, you get busy and forget about that one until it comes to the evening, and that's the biggest problem. It is difficult because you feel good and are not at your home or your office all the time; you are in different places.

One of the reasons Bo was able to live with his cardiac illness for nearly four decades was because of his medications. There is no doubt about it. What's ironic is that the advances in treatment of coronary artery disease really started with coronary surgery, and Bo got two rounds of that. Then, in the last twenty years, there have been rapid advances in preventive medical therapy. Statins were introduced for the first time in the early 1980s. The angiotensin converting enzyme (ACE) inhibitors came out in 1987 and angiotensin receptor blockers in 2001. So Bo was on aspirin, a statin, an ACE inhibitor, and, more recently, the angiotensin receptor blocker (ARB), which slows down kidney disease in diabetes and lowers blood pressure. Bo ended up being the beneficiary of a series of medical treatment advances that came along just at the right time. The other aspect that helped was that Bo sought out advances for each problem. He was never satisfied with the status quo, especially when things weren't going well.

As disciplined as Bo was, even he had an episode where he was home alone a few days and lost track of his medications. His maid found him trying to start his car with the wrong set of keys, and soon Coach Lloyd Carr and some of his staff were there with Bo's cardiologist trying to find out what had happened. He had missed his medications, had not eaten, and got into trouble. Bo recovered from this incident fine, but even a disciplinarian like Bo needed his wife and friends to help him stay on track.

Medications to Treat Heart Disease

A number of medications are helpful in preventing heart disease and its complications. Some prevent or relieve the symptoms of heart disease. Medications commonly prescribed for people at risk for heart disease or having heart disease include:

Beta-blockers slow the heart rate and allow it to beat with less force. They are used to treat high blood pressure and some arrhythmias (abnormal heart rhythms) and help reduce the risk of a repeat heart attack. They can also delay or prevent the development of angina and benefit patients with a weakened heart muscle. Bo was on a beta-blocker for years for all these reasons.

Antiplatelet agents are medications that prevent blood platelets from clumping together to form harmful clots. These medications are used in people who have had a heart attack, have angina, or have had an angioplasty or bypass procedure. Aspirin is one type of antiplatelet medicine. Another is a drug called clopidogrel. For patients who have had a coronary stent placed in an artery or a recent heart attack, both aspirin and clopidogrel are often used together for months, up to a year or more, since their combination is more effective than either one alone.

ACE inhibitors stop the body from producing a protein that narrows blood vessels. These agents are used to treat high blood pressure and have also been shown to benefit patients with a weakened heart muscle. ACE inhibitors also appear to reduce the risk of kidney damage in patients with diabetes. Since Bo had all of these—heart attack, hypertension, weakened heart muscle, diabetes, and mild kidney problems—ACE inhibitors were a critical element of his treatment.

Some patients who take ACE inhibitors develop a dry irritating cough. Thankfully, a similar class of medications without this side effect, called **ARBs (angiotensin receptor blockers)**, have similar benefits of ACE inhibitors for heart muscle damage, preventing progression of kidney failure, and for treating hypertension (or high blood pressure). Bo benefited by taking both of these agents.

There are several types of **cholesterol-lowering drugs**. The most common, **statins**, are used to decrease LDL, or "bad" cholesterol levels in the blood. Other types are used to increase the HDL, or "good," cholesterol and to lower triglycerides. Commonly used cholesterol-lowering medications include bile acid sequestrants, niacin, fibrates, and cholesterol-absorption inhibitors. Bo had taken statins for more than 15 years.

Diuretics (water pills) decrease fluid buildup in the body and are useful in treating high blood pressure. Diuretics can also help to prevent stroke, heart attack, and heart failure. For patients who already have heart failure, diuretics reduce the tendency for fluid buildup in the lungs and swelling in the feet and ankles. Bo used diuretics regularly to reduce his tendency to retain fluid. His dosage and frequency were adjusted frequently based on his daily weight, his blood pressure, and his tendency to retain fluid in his legs, a condition called edema.

Nitrates relax blood vessels. Nitrates in different forms can be used to relieve the discomfort of an angina attack, to prevent an unexpected episode of angina, or to reduce the number of angina episodes that occur over days, weeks, or months by using the medicine regularly on a long-term basis. Bo had angina that was so mild that he rarely needed this medication.

Managing Angina

Angina is chest pain or pressure caused by a temporary lack of oxygen to the heart muscle. In helping Bo manage his angina, he was cautioned in several key areas.

First, he tried to avoid triggers of angina. Anything that makes the heart work harder can cause angina. This includes unusual or extreme physical activity, emotional stress, cold weather, eating a big meal, high blood pressure, being overweight, and cigarette smoking. Bo was especially careful to avoid combined triggers, like going out in cold weather right after eating a heavy meal. A big meal causes the body to devote a larger share of the heart's blood flow to the intestines as the body digests a meal. This actually robs the heart of some of its normal blood flow, thus increasing the risk for angina. Because of his diabetes, Bo tried to eat multiple smaller meals in a day, which also reduced the likelihood of experiencing angina after a meal.

If exercise is a trigger for angina or, worse yet, a heart attack, why did Bo work out nearly every day in order to "nourish" his heart? The answer is complicated, but in its most simple terms, regular exercise helps the heart protect itself.

When Bo exercised each day, his body tended to lose weight so he was closer to ideal body weight. By reducing the fat stores in his body, the control of Bo's diabetes was more consistent and effective. Regular exercise also lowers blood pressure. Regular exercise helps raise levels of healthy HDL cholesterol.

Finally, regular exercise helps the heart learn to develop new blood vessels to areas of heart muscle that are supplied by partially or completely blocked arteries or bypass grafts. In some ways, this is the most miraculous benefit of exercise. Essentially, Bo "auto bypassed" a number of his diseased coronary arteries and old obstructed bypass grafts from his earlier cardiac operations. It is ironic that by stressing the heart with daily walking or bike riding or using Bo's favorite machine, the NuStep, his heart was prompted again and again to form new blood vessels, collateral "detour" arteries, that took up the slack for his old ones! By warming up and cooling down before moderate exercise, the immediate risk of the exercise is reduced, and by doing it regularly, long-term benefits can be realized.

Managing Diabetes

Diabetes was very difficult for Bo, especially late in his life. The neuropathy in his feet prevented him from working out as he had in the past. It made walking the beach in Florida nearly impossible for him. He had to use the NuStep machine while seated. Oftentimes he would be waiting to speak at a banquet and finally, when it was his turn, he could not feel his feet. This numbness made it difficult for him to make it to the podium. All the while the rest of Bo was in good shape, he just could not move his feet very well.

Bo: I remember stages of my own battle to treat my diabetes. Before I went to shots, I made a vow to my endocrinologist, Dr. Jeffrey Sanfield, "Don't you ever ask me to take a shot, because I'm not doing it! You give me those pills and that's it." But soon I couldn't control it.

Can you believe that now I take three or four shots a day! I usually start out the day with a blood sugar between 88 and 110 mg/dL (normal is less than 110 mg/dL). And then I take a shot. I test it again in the afternoon, and if I take my afternoon shot, I just take 10 units. At bedtime I take 50 units of long-acting insulin. Usually I do very nicely with three shots. I don't have to take four very often. I can keep my blood sugar right about 100 mg/dL.

What's next? I have to take all this stuff, but I have gotten used to it now, and I'm still doing it. You know what changed me? I spoke for Rich Hewlett, one of my quarterbacks, at a Childhood Diabetes banquet. Rich has a son, cutest kid you ever saw, good athlete, who has childhood diabetes, and they had a big banquet raising money for childhood diabetes. And they paraded out three or four of the cutest kids you ever saw, all of about 10, 12 years old, and they all had diabetes. And Oh Boy!... Rich told me how his son—he takes four shots a day; I mean, I'm talking about a kid! And I said, "If that young kid can do it, what the hell, I can do it." Now, I try to help raise money for fighting diabetes, too.

Jeffrey Sanfield, Bo's endocrinologist, noted Bo had type 2 diabetes for a long time, probably over 30 years. The term diabetes is usually interchanged with the lay terms

"high blood sugar," "increased blood sugar," "hyperglyce-
mia," or "high blood glucose."

- Diabetes is the third leading cause of death by
  disease.
- Diabetes is growing at an annual rate of approximately
  5 percent, largely due to the increasing average age
  of the population, the increasing rate of obesity, and
  our increasingly sedentary lifestyle. An estimated 16
  million individuals have type 2 diabetes in the United
  States.
- Compared with non-diabetic persons, patients with
  diabetes are two to six times more likely to have a
  stroke; 25 times more prone to blindness; twice as
  likely to suffer heart attacks; 17 times more prone to
  kidney disease; and five times more likely to incur
  gangrene (diabetes accounts for 40–45 percent of all
  non-traumatic amputations annually).

Millions of people have it and many don't know they
have it because they are relatively asymptomatic. The
term "relatively asymptomatic" is often used because many
patients may not attribute the symptoms they have to diabetes. For example, fatigue is a common symptom but the
fatigue is not specific for diabetes. The classic symptoms
of diabetes are: Excessive thirst, frequent need to urinate,
poor wound healing, and blurred vision. Through the years
that Bo fought diabetes, he rarely complained of symptomatic diabetes, which makes identifying and treating diabetes even more difficult.

Bo started like most patients using the most common drug treatment agents, specifically sulfonylureas
(glimepiride, glipizide, glyburide). Sulfonylureas *stimu-
late* the pancreas to make extra insulin and, combined
with diet and exercise, were the cornerstone of Bo's initial

treatment. Bo, like many patients, had to work hard on his diet. People with diabetes have to limit carbohydrates, particularly simple sugars. An example of a simple sugar is a candy bar or a nondiet (i.e., not sugar-free) bottle of soda pop. Bo had no trouble avoiding these types of foods because he did not consider them a mainstay of his diet. However, like many patients, watching portion size and carbohydrates was difficult for him, because he spent a great deal of his time traveling, as someone's guest, or speaking at dinner banquets. He attended many fund-raisers and social functions that inherently led to problems in portion size and choice.

Many patients with type 2 diabetes try to eat right, exercise, and use one pill. They hope to avoid the move to either more pills or even insulin. Unfortunately, the natural progression of diabetes, even for those who eat right and exercise, often necessitates the move to insulin, as over time the pancreas begins to lose more function. Following a strict diet may slow the progress of diabetes, but it may not be enough to stop its progression.

Bo's greatest strength in managing his diabetes was his passion for exercise. In fact, when he could not exercise he probably felt most stressed and most unhealthy. He would often express at his visits to his endocrinologist, Jeff Sanfield, some of his concerns for the weight and the health issues of his players. The life expectancy of a professional football player had dropped to 56 years. He noticed that many of them had become overweight, especially the offensive linemen. When former Ohio State and Minnesota Viking offensive lineman Kory Stringer died of heat exhaustion following practice, Bo reflected that the linemen of today had become too heavy. When he coached offensive linemen, they were smaller than current college and NFL standards, and Bo felt that many of the athletes of today, and some of his previous players, were no longer well-conditioned, but rather simply overweight. Bo became very sensitive to this because of the implications of being overweight to his own health and his diabetes.

In Bo's case, although he exercised and ate as carefully as possible, his pancreas began to lose function over time and he was no longer able to manage it with a simple drug like glyburide. Dr. Sanfield prescribed to Bo the medication metformin, another popular anti-diabetic drug that helps one's own insulin work better. However, because of gastrointestinal side effects and reduced kidney function (later in Bo's life), this drug could no longer be used. Also, some drugs used to treat diabetes can have adverse drug interactions with heart medications. For example, an oral agent for diabetes treatment might cause liver inflammation when combined with a cholesterol medication such as a statin. Thus, Bo and his doctors, as a team, were very careful to consider such potential interactions as his treatment evolved, as well as monitoring his liver- and kidney-function blood tests.

Diabetics monitor their blood glucose level by pricking their finger with a monitoring device called a glucose monitor. The target for blood sugar control changed through the years Bo had diabetes. A fasting blood sugar of 126 mg/dL or less was considered within normal limits when Bo was diagnosed. Now fasting blood sugars over 100 are considered a concern. Post-eating blood glucoses should generally run less than 140 mg/dL. Bo's blood glucose control was also monitored at periodic doctor visits with a test referred to as a hemoglobin A_1C, which is a measure of how well the diabetes has been controlled over several months. This allows the patient and physician to have insight as to how their control has been during periods of time when they may not have been checking their blood glucose.

Bo, like many patients, experienced complications from diabetes. It was probably the link between diabetes and heart disease that ultimately took his life. Diabetes contributes to hardening of the arteries, also known as coronary disease as outlined in other portions of this book.

Diabetes also contributes to nerve damage, referred to as neuropathy, such that the lower extremities, i.e., legs, lose sensation. In Bo's case, this contributed to less mobility later in life and nerve pain. As part of managing his diabetic neuropathy, Bo was under the care of a neurologist and took medications to reduce the pain from nerve damage. The neuropathy was a particular source of unpleasantness to Bo, not from just the pain standpoint, but because it limited his exercise, his strength, and ability to walk. The public expected Bo Schembechler to be strong, and any appearance of frailness in his ability to walk was particularly disturbing to him. As he got older, his ability to remain vibrant and active became important to Bo. Quality of life and the ability to do the things he enjoyed became increasingly important. As the complications gradually took hold, Bo chose not to complain or express a "why me" attitude. His approach was always to see what he could do to impact what was occurring in a positive way. Eating right and trying to exercise more were always steps that Bo had in his control and he implemented them daily. Over the years with diabetes, heart disease, and high cholesterol, Bo was frustrated by the multiple medications he had to take. However, he dealt with this frustration in a constructive way, challenging his care team to make sure that each medication had a clear purpose and checking to ensure that any possible unfavorable interaction was being considered.

The most difficult aspect of diabetes that Bo struggled with was checking his blood sugars on a consistent basis.

The pricking of one's finger four times a day and then taking a shot of insulin to adjust the blood glucose level was not easy. For years Bo used a plan that involved three to four shots a day. He would take a shot of long-acting insulin at bedtime and then he would combine it with two or three shots of short-acting insulin with meals during the day. Occasionally, when he was out and busy, he would omit a shot, and as he got older his needs changed in the amount of insulin he required. When he ate less, he would obviously take less insulin, and when he was more active he would also reduce his dose. His blood glucose averages through the years were remarkably good considering his hectic lifestyle and schedule. His three-month average Hb A_1C level was often below 7 percent, which would put his blood sugars on the favorable average of 100 to 150 mg/dL. On rare occasions, such as when he was ill or omitted a shot, he would have very high blood sugar. If Bo exercised more than usual, he might have a drop in his blood sugar. He managed the swings when they occurred with the same matter-of-factness that he handled other aspects of his life and medical conditions—with immediate attention.

Managing diabetes and its complications is no small task. As Dr. Sanfield found: "Bo had specialists in eye disease, neurology, kidney disease, heart disease, joint disease, diabetes, and peripheral vascular disease to help him manage his problems and anticipate future issues."

Bo was always able to assemble a team of health care providers that supported and reflected his spirit, perseverance, and, most of all, willingness to work together as a team. Like the complex game of football with specialty coaches, managing diabetes and related complications requires the assembly of a team of medical specialists that best meets the patient's needs. If Bo had any message to tell other patients with diabetes, it would be to (1) do what you need to do to take care of yourself and (2) assemble a team that will help support those aspects of care that are required.

In addition to his medical doctors, Bo's wife Cathy was clearly a major component of his success over the last thirteen years of his life. She attended crucial clinic visits when Bo was not feeling well, and she was always available to help support any aspect of care that Bo needed. She provided that extra motivation he needed at times when he was weary of fighting a chronic disease like diabetes. As his health gradually declined over the last several years, her support became even more valuable. The term *team* as it applies to diabetes treatment includes family members who can see the daily subtleties of the disease that are so important to monitor and be there when a loved one needs them.

The Fourth Quarter— 2003–2006

Something Isn't Right!

Bo's passion for living never wavered, but there were times when he knew he was in trouble. His heart function was significantly compromised by the heart attacks. Part of his heart just did not work very well at all. As he battled cardiovascular disease through his life, there always seemed to be a medical answer to his need when he needed it. Bo would spend more time in the hospital taking advantage of medical enhancements and getting "tuned up" during the fourth quarter of his life.

Bo: For some reason, I never lost my confidence that I would not give up fighting my medical problems. Well, there was one exception just before my pacemaker was put in when I really felt bad. I thought that maybe the heart muscle was getting tired. I mean, it has taken a real beating, and you know, it's just coming to a point where maybe it's not going to be able to function any longer. And that's what I thought, I knew I felt bad, and I was not myself.

I couldn't walk. My legs were like heavy weights. And the darndest thing was how episodic it was. I would have a great day and then I'd have a lousy day, and I couldn't figure out what in the world is doing this. But it was especially bad at night. My legs would hurt like you couldn't believe!

Finally, one night in November of 2004, Cathy checked my pulse during a bad spell of leg pain and it was 30 beats a minute! I went to the hospital and the next thing I knew they put in a pacemaker.

Gary Moeller remembers when Bo received the pacemaker and the difference it made. "I was supposed to go see Bo because he was complaining about having to have this pacemaker, and so I call him up and he says, 'This is the darndest thing in the world, Mo! Now they got them where if it's too high, I make a phone call and they fix it over the phone! This is the neatest thing I've ever done. You can't believe this, Mo.' And then he started telling me the whole story. He was so excited to have this pacemaker. His heart beat was real low, and this treatment helped control it. Mentally it really fixed him up. Now he was all positive on how great pacemakers are.

"I told him, 'You were just crying about this last week.' He says, 'Oh, I did not!' Then he'd laugh like hell, you know, oh he loved getting that pacemaker. It just seemed like it put life in him. Just like it pumped him up and gave him some spark. Yeah, it was like it pumped new life into him. He was really darn right excited about that thing."

Lloyd Carr visited Bo and describes the visit: "Bo was not doing well and they put him in the hospital. So I went to see him and he says, 'You have got to see this,' and he puts on this video of how a pacemaker worked. It was really interesting, but he was studying what he was getting into!

"He wasn't feeling well at all. That was on a Friday and then the pacemaker was put in. Monday, he came into the office, he's dancing around. He's telling everybody he is a new man. He said, 'It's unbelievable how I feel, this is a miracle.' He just kept fighting. He always rallied."

Mary Passink was amazed at the difference. "You would have thought he was five years younger. He looked and acted like he was five years younger!"

Bo's Heart Disease Complications

When he was feeling bad, Bo assumed that he had developed a weak heart. Congestive heart failure is a condition in which the heart cannot pump out enough blood to supply the body's needs, and blood tends to build up "in" and "behind" the heart itself. Affecting millions of Americans, heart failure occurs when excess fluid collects in the body as a result of heart stiffness, weakness, injury, abnormalities of the heart's valve functions, and/or irregularities of the heart's rhythm. High blood pressure is a leading cause of congestive heart failure. Coronary heart disease and diabetes are also major underlying causes of heart failure. Remarkably, Bo had not one but four of the underlying causes for heart failure: an arrhythmia, coronary heart disease, hypertension, and diabetes.

Arrhythmias are problems that affect the electrical system of the heart muscle, producing an abnormal beating of the heart. Arrhythmias are interruptions in the normal sequence of the heart's pumping action. Many problems can cause arrhythmias, including coronary artery disease, thyroid imbalance, high blood pressure, diabetes, smoking, heavy alcohol use, an electrolyte imbalance, drug abuse, and stress. Certain medicines and dietary supplements such as ephedra can also cause cardiac arrhythmias.

A very common arrhythmia is called **atrial fibrillation**, which affects millions of Americans. It is more common in older people and those with acquired heart diseases such as hypertension, coronary heart disease, and valvular heart disease. Atrial fibrillation occurs when the heart's upper two of its four chambers (the atria) quiver or fibrillate instead of beating in unison with the lower chambers (the ventricles). When this happens, blood isn't pumped completely out of the atria, making it more likely to pool and clot. If a clot breaks free from the heart and becomes lodged in an artery in the brain, a stroke results. About 15 percent of strokes are caused by atrial fibrillation. Clots may also travel to other areas of the body, the most common to the arteries in the thigh and knee regions.

Bo: Another challenge I had was occasionally my heart was beating like the dickens. I didn't know how fast it was beating, but I knew it wasn't right. I also noticed that my legs started to swell and I had more trouble doing my bicycle exercise. I went to my cardiologist and he describes this treatment where they go up through the groin and they zap the bad circuit in your heart, and that lets the electrical system work normally again. My arrhythmia went away for good. I couldn't believe it!

A close cousin to atrial fibrillation is **atrial flutter**. In this arrhythmia, the upper chambers of the heart beat at a very fast rate (e.g., 300 times per minute). The lower main pumping chambers of the heart (the ventricles) can't beat this fast, but they often will beat at 100 times or even 150 times per minute. When Bo developed atrial flutter, he noticed both acceleration in his heart action as well as signs of congestive heart failure (shortness of breath and accumulation of fluid [edema] in the ankles and lower leg regions). He underwent a procedure where the abnormal electrical circuit was interrupted using a special procedure called catheter-based ablation. This cured Bo of his atrial flutter.

Development of an abnormally slow heart rhythm, **bradycardia**, can also complicate coronary heart disease. In Bo's case, compromised blood supply injured the heart area where his natural pacemaker resided and controlled the electrical impulses of his heart. This slow rhythm was intermittent and was especially prominent at night. He was thinking his heart muscle was shot and he was on his last legs. Finally, during a particularly lousy night, Cathy checked his blood pressure and pulse, identifying a severe reduction in both. His nearly miraculous response to receiving an artificial pacemaker confirmed that much of his recent deterioration wasn't heart failure or angina, but rather his failing natural pacemaker.

How to Juggle Multiple Medications

Patients who see multiple physicians need to take charge of the medications they are being given. Bo was used to running a team and he demanded the same from his physicians as he did from his team. They had to have clear communication so all knew what play was being called. Bo demanded to know what each medication he was taking would do and how it might react with his other medications. Likewise, he wanted all his physicians to communicate with each other on what they were prescribing, so all were on the same page.

Bo: I have always worried about interaction of pills, because I put these pills in my stomach, and they all run together. I just wonder sometimes if there is a bad chemical reaction. But, since I know the medicines have a purpose, I just make sure all of my docs know what I am taking.

There are more times after you have taken medicine, or after you have worked out, that you feel good, than there are times that you feel bad. So you are going for those times that feel good, and you do the things necessary to make you feel good. Now you can feel bad if you want to, I mean, just start neglecting all these things, and you will feel bad. But, you know, it's like healthy guys that work out, after they work out, they feel good. Well, I do too. After I eat, take a shower, man I feel good, and so there are more times when you feel good than when you feel bad. And so you're shooting for as many times to feel good as you can. That will give you discipline.

Coordination of prescription medicines is critical. Many Americans are being treated by multiple doctors, each prescribing different medications. This is a recipe for disaster! Bo had one doctor write his prescriptions and this physician was in close communication with his other doctors. Bo got all of his medications from the same pharmacy. This minimized the chance of error.

Bo was seeing an orthopedist, cardiologist, neurologist, surgeon, rheumatologist, and a diabetes specialist! It was very important that Bo's physicians communicated effectively and shared medical records, which in his case, while at different medical centers, was relatively easy since they practiced together in a single community.

One of the biggest problems with healthcare in general is that the doctors are not on the same page. When Bo formed his medical team, the doctors couldn't mess things up. If they did, he would change the team. He had high expectations and he was careful to be sure his team didn't get sloppy.

Tips for Taking Medications

"Take your medicine." It sounds simple, but there can be a lot to remember when you take regular medication—especially if you're taking many of them. Here are some tips that have helped patients like Bo.

- Bo placed "sticky notes" or simple medication lists in visible places to remind him to take the medicines. Notes on the refrigerator, on the bathroom mirror, or on the inside of the front door, especially when Cathy was away, were helpful to him.
- Bo used a weekly pill box with separate compartments (available at most drugstores). He kept the box in a key spot where he saw it when he went about his daily routine. Bo had a very disciplined strategy for filling, using, and tracking his pill intake using this weekly pill box.
- Bo used a pill calendar to remind himself when he needed a refill.
- Some patients wear a wristwatch with an alarm. This is especially helpful to remind patients about medications, like insulin, to be taken during busy times of the day.

Monitoring the Effects of Medical Treatment

Managing chronic medical conditions like angina, hypertension, heart failure, and diabetes takes tremendous discipline and daily monitoring of bodily functions. Bo Schembechler did this as well as anyone. He checked his weight, blood sugar, blood pressure, and pulse. He wrote his readings in a diary so he could track changes over time. When a number was out of line, he contacted his doctors to explore what might be going on and what to do. He recognized over the years that a person's medical condition was not static, but rather dynamic. Depending on food and fluid intake, humidity, exercise, salt intake, stress, and other factors, health status can change from day to day or week to week.

Bo was the greatest patient for a cardiologist to have. He would call his cardiologist and say, "My blood pressure's up. Something's not right." Care teams need to know about problems as soon as they are identified so they are caught before they become difficult to treat.

Too often we hear from patients that they do not want to bother anyone, especially when it is late at night or on a weekend. In reality, healthcare providers need timely notification that something is not right to aid patients to win their battle. Too often a delay will take the opportunity to help out of physicians' hands, and then there are no winners. For example, Michigan's former athletic director Don Canham knew something was wrong in his abdomen, but waited 12 hours and died enroute to his doctor's office of a leaking aneurysm. Your caregivers are there to help you, but you must help them in doing their job.

The Role of Attitude and
Staying Focused when You're Down

Health problems can wear us down, and even defeat us before our time, if we let them. Bo had a wonderful outlook on life that permitted him to appreciate every day, even though some were a lot better than others. His desire to be there for others, to make a difference in tomorrow, and then to be there for his partner Cathy motivated him to keep a positive attitude.

Bo: Through my various problems, I have been down at times, but I don't know if I have been depressed. I always felt like there's something that I could do. You get up in the morning, you look out there, the sun is shining, the birds are singing, and sure as the sun rises my players are calling me to check in. I was never about records to be broken, so that was never a disappointment to me. Cripe ... my players kept me busy all day with letters, phone calls, stopping in to visit.

I might be hurting inside, but I never really can say I was depressed. After my heart attack in 1969, I always thought I was going to make it back to coaching. I have been blessed to feel like I am on a mission, which was not about breaking records or being in the limelight. A mission to make a difference in the lives of young people in some way has kept me motivated to keep going.

Bo's attitude may have been his greatest strength. When all around were "down" or disappointed, Bo always seemed to have that vision of what needed to be done and went about taking on challenges and fixing the problem. But Bo, too, had times when his attitude wasn't the asset it usually was. One of the most telling times came in late 2002 when friend and former player Fritz Seyferth visited Bo. He was not himself; he was "down." Bo thought he had hit the end of the road for his heart care. Was the end approaching? He could not fathom it. He was down, but said he was going to get suggestions on what could be done. Fritz had just started working with the University of Michigan Cardiovascular Center and suggested Bo take a look there. After a long conversation where Bo expressed "I am just not ready to be put out to pasture," they walked to Bo's car and Bo asked Fritz, "What do you think I should do?"

Fritz responded, "The first thing you can do is fix your attitude!"

To which Bo responded, "You think that is what I need? Well, I can do that!"

You could see the fight in Bo's eyes, as he had a challenge and he was getting game ready to beat this opponent. And Bo made an appointment to see Dr. Eagle at the University of Michigan's Cardiovascular Center that next week. He never sought further advice. He knew he had found a team of people who would give him all the resources he needed to fight his battle with cardiovascular disease. He trusted the team completely—not that he stopped interrogating each caregiver to be sure they knew exactly what they were doing!

Depression and Coronary Heart Disease

Study after study has confirmed that depression occurs commonly after people suffer a heart attack or undergo coronary bypass surgery. In addition, these same studies confirm that the presence of depression creates a greater risk for future complications. This is probably related to several factors. Patients who are depressed tend to be less successful in reaching their dietary and exercise goals. They may be less compliant with their medications, have reduced success with stopping smoking, and skip their follow-up doctor visits. And finally, apart from all of these effects, depression itself seems to be related to the triggering of heart attacks and other complications. For all these reasons, identifying and treating a patient's depression after a heart attack and a major heart procedure is a top priority. Bo's tendencies to feel "down" after several of his cardiac events were short-lived and not recurrent.

Bo: I can honestly say to you that the reason I loved coaching was because I love players ... 17- to 22-year-old guys, I can sit down and talk to them. Players, that's the difference, and that's my product. That is what I deal in. Some guys build gadgets; I try to build people. Steelcase Chairman Jimmy Hackett has adopted one of my practices: Anytime one of his employees, and he has tens of thousands, wants to talk, he stops whatever he is doing to listen and talk ... He says, "Not that many people come in. I always feel once I get them in there, I learn more about what's going on down in the factory than talking to my supervisors." He learned that from me, that you have an open-door policy—just let them come in—and it has surfaced a lot of potential problems that never went any further. I loved those meetings.

Involvement in this medical care and coaching kept Bo active, involved with others, and seeking knowledge. Lloyd Carr describes Bo's interaction with staff: "One of the beautiful things about him, he never blamed anybody, he wasn't looking to point the finger, he was always trying to find a solution. He would challenge you all the time. He would ask. 'Why are you playing so-and-so?' and you had to defend what you were doing. And in the process of defending your decision, sometimes you came to the realization that he really wanted to make sure you had thought this through. And in defending your position, sometimes you found it was not as strong as you had thought it was and you wound up giving somebody else a chance. He challenged us in everything we did. 'Why are you recruiting this kid?' It never ended!

"As a staff, we would have unbelievable fights about everything from politics to baseball, screaming and yelling. Those staff meetings were fun, you were energized and on your game or you would be crucified. On the outside, he had this reputation of being a tyrant, but he liked disagreement. He liked conflict, because when you have open and honest arguments, you really find out what people think and sometimes you learn something. He was very inquisitive, and he had a lot of interest outside of football and that's what made him fun to be around."

Kim Eagle relates that "He methodically challenged every medicine I've started or stopped. Every visit, he wanted to know, 'Why am I on this?' When we started talking about writing this book he'd say, 'Why are you doing this?'"

Overtime—2006

Bo and His Doctors—Creating a Winning Team

Bo Schembechler recognized after his first heart attack and other heart complications that having an effective partnership with his care team was essential to creating a winning game plan. There were several facets to his approach from which others can learn.

- Bo took ownership of his care; he *spoke up*!
- Bo understood what it meant to be a *good patient.* He was completely honest in answering questions that his doctors had and open in identifying areas of his care plans that either were not working well or where he was falling down. He told doctors that he wanted to stop the heart disease from getting worse and would like help in achieving that goal. He asked about the latest advances in controlling his disease including its risk factors, how to maximize his lifestyle goals, and how to have the best combination of medications to improve his chances.
- Bo understood exercise and diet, the essential components of his medical game plan. His lifestyle goals included exercising at least 30 minutes a day, not overeating, choosing foods that were not high in fat or sugar wherever possible, avoiding tobacco, and limiting his alcohol use to a minimum.

- He made sure to understand when his next appointment would be and what to do in the event of new or concerning signs or symptoms.
- When things were not going well or he was concerned with his care or response to it, Bo brought his wife to the appointment to ensure that his questions were gone over and answered.

Rudy Reichert knows that "Bo was always smart about making sure his medical game plan was clear. It was his nature. He was always testing to see if we were going the right way. It was like, 'Have I got the right contractor, the right plumber, the right doctor?' "

Bo: I listened to my doctors. I'd go in there and listen. They'd tell me what they think. My doctors never said, "You have to do this, you have to do that." They didn't do that. It was, "Well, probably you should do this." So then I would just take whatever they said and I would do it.

I have always had confidence that I had the best possible medical attention. I had doctors who were interested in me. They always took care of me. For any patient, I'd say make sure that you have total confidence in the doctors you are dealing with. Because if you do not, I don't think you will do the things that are necessary. If you don't have that confidence, you should make a change. Man, my life's important. I've got to find a doctor that I have confidence in.

There is a chemistry that has to happen with a doctor and a patient. That has a lot to do with whether they will have the spirit to fight this disease every day. And if you don't have confidence, you probably won't follow their advice. So I say, don't be afraid to make a change in your medical team if you have uncertainties. Get second opinions if you're facing a big decision. You've got to be confident that your game plan is right for you.

Don't think that because you're not a celebrity that you can't get proper treatment from good doctors, and the latest treatments you may not know anything about. Science is changing everyday; they are making advances all the time. People need to understand how, by seeking expert advice, they will benefit. I can see some people being reluctant. You have to pursue it. I can see some guy saying, "Oh, I don't want to go up there and bother anybody." That's a mistake ... don't feel that way!

Bo's confidence in his medical care was built on trust, and part of that trust was the idea that a game plan isn't unilateral: it is the development of a consensus. He would ask, "Tell me again, what's this medicine for?" He sought caregivers who were open to being challenged. He recognized that this was a give and take.

Bo wasn't afraid to change. In a way, this is like the game planning he'd do with his coaches before a big game. He'd challenge the defensive scheme, the offensive game plan, always probing, looking for weaknesses in the plan. In approaching his medical care this way, he had complete confidence that the game plan was right.

Bo: No, I've made no mistakes. That's the way I look at it. In whom I've dealt with, the medicines I take, the things I've done, I've made no mistakes. Now you might look at me and say, "You could have done better if you'd done this or that," but you know, in the position I'm in right now, and the way I feel right now, there were no mistakes. It's interesting, I know people who go to their doctors and when they go, I say, "Let me go with you to meet this guy." I may be dead wrong, but I've always felt that I could judge people pretty well. So when I met a doctor, and asked a few questions, then I'd come out of there and tell my friend, "I think you're okay there," or "I think, better look around and get somebody else!"

What makes good doctors? Can I trust what they say? Are they really interested in answering my questions for my benefit? Do they listen? Do they seem to be confident in their knowledge? Do they communicate in a way that I can understand? Do they inspire confidence in me that I would be able to respond to them? Do I feel like I am one of a hundred patients, or do I feel like I am the only one? I may be one of a hundred, but right now, you and me, I'm the one." That's what I want to feel.

My football team was only as good as the last play, the last game, or the last player, the last guy. Say I have 125 guys on my team: that 125th guy is important, or he shouldn't be on the team. He's important because if I have to have a guy impersonate the other opponent's center, and that 125th guy does that, I want him to bust his tail to do whatever it is he can to make us better, because if he does that, we have a better chance to win. I always did this and it may not have always looked like it, but I was interested in every player. I didn't want any player coming in there with a bad attitude. If he's the 125th guy, I'm not going to say, "Oh, who gives a darn, he's just the 125th guy anyway." That's what allowed me to be so hard on the players, because they knew, number one that I cared. And when I'm looking at a doctor I want to make sure that this doctor cares.

You have to look at a doctor just like you do anybody else you deal with. That doctor's dealing with other problems with other patients and they have got a lot on their platter. But they still need to be able to zero in on me for just a few minutes when I look at them, and say,

"They are really interested in my problem here." Isn't that right? That's what makes the difference.

Getting the right medical team in place helps with your attitude. I have changed doctors. I had to. I needed a team that would say, "Coach, here's the game plan and you have got to carry the ball!" We all need hope and a team that creates an atmosphere of hope.

Beyond the Medical Team

The importance of the role of a spouse or other health advocate cannot be over emphasized in the impact it has on the quality and quantity of life when we are in the fourth quarter. Bo had his personal patient advocate in Cathy. She monitored how he was doing continually and got him the care he needed on a timely basis. Otherwise, Bo may not have been as proactive. Now a day hardly goes by for Cathy Schembechler that some acquaintance of Bo's doesn't thank her for all she did, allowing Bo to give his community more years than any thought they would get.

Bo: Sometimes I might not want to bother my doctors, and my wife would say, "You know, Bo, this is across the line. You ought to just be sure here; we need to make a phone call." A good partner is important in medical care. It helps you sort out when things are working well, and when they aren't. You gain another more objective opinion.

In that episode where my pulse got really low, I can tell you, I would not have gone to the hospital until the next morning, but Cathy would not let me go back to bed! She knew I needed to go to the hospital. She also helped me with planning advances in my treatment plan. She read a lot and checked things out in medical books or online. And when it was something that affected us, it was worthwhile to look it up. We all need to be doing that—she just did it better than me, and I am grateful.

Cathy gave me the insulin shots when she was around. She was very good at it, but we've got these needles that are a little too long right now, I think they go all the way to the bone! When I do the injections, she kind of looks over my shoulder to be sure I am doing the right things.

Anybody that is in the position that I am in and has a healthy relationship with their spouse—that is money in the bank. Believe me, that is money in the bank. When I was moping around after Millie died, before I met Cathy, I didn't know where I was going to end up. You have more to fight for when you have a relationship like I've had. When you have somebody that you love, and you want that person to be happy, you want to stay alive, and you've just got to keep it going. That is what I feel, and I'm not trying to be sentimental about it, I'm just saying that's why I am like I am; because I don't think I'd be here without her. Her support is vital with all the challenges I have, she keeps me going. I need her leading my team.

Many patients like Bo recognize how critical it is to have a spouse or other advocate to help them stay on track. Whether it's checking medication use, watching for early signs of deterioration, or helping achieve diet, exercise, and other goals, a health advocate or coach helps heart patients stay focused and on track. First Millie, and more recently Cathy, helped Bo enormously. Without them, it seems unlikely that he'd have lived as long as he did.

Bo's secretary and assistant heard him express these feelings. Mary Passink stated, "Bo's sheer determination and will to live were instrumental in his fight against his heart disease. Cathy had a lot to do with his desire to live. Just yesterday he was getting ready to leave the office, he said, 'And I hope I have lots of years with this gal yet.' "

Lynn Koch, Bo's assistant, believes that "Cathy was real good about keeping him on the level with his diet and his lifestyle. She had to step up and be firm when Bo got going, speaking all over the place all times of night, because that was when he got out of his routine and got worn out. When asked with Cathy at his side 'What motivates you to keep your discipline to fight your cardiovascular disease,' Bo replied, with tears welling in his eyes, 'I want to have as much time with this wonderful gal next to me as I can. We are good for each other.' "

The Two-Minute Drill

While football is a game and cardiovascular disease is life and death, having a plan in place to handle the sudden situations you are put in is critical for victory in both cases.

College football practice covers all phases of the game to be played on a Saturday. Teams work on the two-minute drill in case the team finds itself behind and needing to score to win the game in the last two minutes.

The medical profession plans for this situation in the life of patients. End of life brings the same challenges. You need to be prepared to achieve the best possible outcome and prevent premature death. Bo did this ... to a degree.

Getting his estate in order was not as difficult as agreeing to an "End of Life—No Herculean Acts" document (Advance Health Care Directive). Bo had a good team of attorneys aid him in preparing his estate plan, and he had that in order when the end finally came. But his personal conviction that "what the mind can conceive and believe the body will achieve" prevented him from signing an End of Life document that would prevent Herculean efforts to save his life.

This was clearly exemplified in a September 2006 hospitalization for congestive heart failure. Bo had gained 17 pounds in fluid weight. Not feeling well, he was admitted to the hospital to reduce the extra body fluid and adjust his heart medications. When Bo was well on his way to recovery, a nurse entered his room and said, "We have a problem, Mr. Schembechler. When you were admitted in July you noted that you had an 'End of Life' agreement. When we admitted you this time, you said that you did not. Do you or do you not have one?"

Bo replied, "I have lots of attorneys and papers, what do you need?"

The nurse explained, "We need to know if you want us to use all means possible to keep you alive, if the need arises?"

Bo resoundingly responded, "You are damn right I do!"

Cathy was sitting at Bo's side and jumped in and said, "Well, I signed an End of Life agreement and I do not want you to do that for me."

Bo turned to Cathy with a look of "I could never let you go" and said, "You will not have anything to say about that if I am around to have a say!"

The week before Bo passed away, Bo and Fritz Seyferth spent the afternoon with Bo's 1971 Rose Bowl quarterback Tom Slade and his family. After a prolonged battle with bone cancer and leukemia, Tom was taken off life support and arrangements were made for Tom to go home with hospice. In this circumstance, Bo saw what the "end of life" looked like in a new way. Bo had been through this with his first wife Millie and other friends, but this was different. This hit home. Bo had felt the responsibility to be there for Tom like a father would have been, as both of Tom's parents were deceased. Bo even returned to Ann Arbor for a week to be with Tom in the hospital the previous winter, when Tom's bone cancer was taking a toll. Seeing Tom unresponsive, his wife trying to hold the family together as his sons tried to communicate with Tom through their tears took a toll on Bo. Yet Bo caressed Tom's arm as he tried to communicate words of support and comfort to Tom, as the minister tried to comfort all. It was very emotional.

Tom's wife Pam had been sleeping in Tom's hospital room and had not eaten. So seven days before Bo's passing, Bo took Pam and Fritz for a late lunch in the hospital cafeteria. Pam described how Tom had made all the preparations for the family and her. Tom had left caring notes in the cupboards, in the dresser, in the closets saying, "If you are doing this I must be in the hospital, so here is some money to take care of things."

Tom had planned his funeral, a life celebration party, and paid for all of it. The detail to which Tom prepared for end of life was remarkable and as Pam so aptly said, "That is so Tom, he planned for everything!"

After Pam went back to Tom's room, Fritz and Bo stayed and talked. Fritz suggested to Bo that if he did not want to think about what it would be like for Cathy and others when he was not around, as Tom had, that was okay, as they discussed the virtues of "What the mind can conceive and believe, the body will achieve." When the talk was concluding, Bo leaned across the table, looked at Fritz straight in the eye, and said, "I am not going to die!!"

Bo attended Tom's funeral the day before he passed away himself.

Beating the Odds—How Bo Did It

The fight in the fourth quarter when we are behind and the clock is running down is the fight for life, and Bo showed all of us how to win the game when the odds were all against him. His is a story of a passion for living from which we all can grow.

Lloyd Carr, who worked with Bo as an assistant coach for nine years, learned from his example. "The first word that comes to my mind is his integrity, and that I think is exemplified in his coaching, the way he conducted his program, and in his life. He is a guy that was extremely honest with his players and his coaches. You knew when you were dealing with him that you were dealing with a guy who was honest and that you could trust. That single quality stands out. I've seen him in situations where he could have bent the rules. He maybe would have won more games, and I don't think there is any doubt that he could have won national championships had he been willing to do some things in recruiting that he refused to compromise on. Then he was a great competitor, he was going to fight to win, he was willing to do all the things that allowed him to be successful. He didn't want to lose. There's the concept of fearing failure and the joy he got from winning. And then, he was an extremely hard worker. Nobody was going to out work him. He said to me one time, 'A lot of people ask me why I work so hard, and why I work all of these long hours. Man, I'm trying to support my family!' And he would talk about his father and what a hard working guy he was.

"Another of his attributes goes right to competitiveness; he was as tough as anybody I've ever known. Bo had this kidney stone and he's in unbelievable pain. It's like having a knife in your side. It is game week and he doesn't miss a meeting, he doesn't miss a practice, and the game is at home, and he's in excruciating pain. It is halftime and we head up the tunnel and Bo and I are at the urinal together and it's obvious he's in pain, and I look down and he's urinating blood. I'll never forget this as long as I live; there are not many as mentally tough as he was.

"The bigger the game, the more controlled and the better he was. We were playing Miami and they had a great team. We had a good lead, but they came back late to beat us. It was a heartbreaking game. There were so many things that happened in the last few minutes of that game that went against us, so it really hurt to lose when it looked like we had a win. So we are headed up the tunnel after a terrible loss and every coach and player is dreading what Bo is going to say, because he hated to lose.

"We get into the locker room, and he says, 'We're going to have a great team, men! We are going to win the Big Ten championship, and go to the Rose Bowl.' We were all taken back, but you know what? That's exactly what we did. At a critical point he said the right thing, and it made all of the difference.

"He was an enemy of complacency. When we had just won a big game and had a 'sure win' the next week, it was hell. There was little anyone could do that week that was done well enough. He was relentless in his command of your attitude. He knew when and how to get you to be mentally ready for the next game."

Jon Falk realizes that "Bo had two great qualities that would help anybody in living, especially if you have a heart issue. First, he could compartmentalize his issues. He could take an issue, focus on it, and once that issue was successfully addressed, then he would move on. He never let things linger a long time, with the exception of the time in 1973 when the Big Ten Athletic Directors voted to choose Ohio State over Michigan to go to the Rose Bowl. That has lingered with him a little bit! If you ever want to get him mad, just ask him about that vote!

"The second quality that he had was that Bo could laugh at himself. If he made a mistake, or if he did something to laugh about, he would laugh at it himself as much as anyone. He had a wonderful sense of humor that revitalized him."

President Gerald Ford reflected on Bo's "wonderful gift of dedication and discipline. I am sure when he began to realize he had a problem, he started down a path of disciplined effort to address it, just like he did every Saturday in preparation for his opponents on the football field.

"Bo's mental outlook was so positive, I think he really believed the mind can heal the body, and it worked for him very well ... and science has evolved in a timely manner for both of us! My relationship with Bo was wonderful. I always enjoyed addressing the Michigan Team and taking what little time we had to talk. He was there when I called on him, and I hope I have been there for him. I know we had a ball in raising the monies needed to build the 'Center of Champions,' now Schembechler Hall. And Bo helped me on some of my fund-raising projects. He was a man of his word, and you cannot say much better about a person."

Kim Eagle, Bo's cardiologist, notes, "He was a walking miracle. If you looked at the blood flow to his heart through these various bypasses that Otto Gago concocted, you would say that his heart muscle should not be alive. All but one of the major arteries were blocked, and what we call collateral blood vessels were coming in from God knows where, heaven I suppose, that were nourishing his heart. It was astonishing."

Understanding Bo's Greatness

"How can people say 'I am having a bad day,' how can you have a bad day?" Later in life Bo made this statement many times, and he would follow it by saying "Just think of how beautiful it is outside, the birds, the trees, and the chance to be in touch with others you care about, to help them if they need it. I do not understand how you can have a bad day." This is the attitude that helped Bo fight his cardiovascular disease so well.

Socrates, Aristotle, and Plato studied why we do what we do and found "Happiness" at the root of our actions. Bo is a marvelous example of the writings of Fr. Robert Spitzer in *The Spirit of Leadership,* where he organizes the findings of Socrates, Aristotle, and Plato on this subject.

Fr. Spitzer writes that we each have four levels of happiness in us, and we need to understand which one of them is driving us most of the time. Bo developed a mature search for happiness as he tried to live his life at the highest level, which Fr. Spitzer defines as Happiness Level 4: "Being involved with something of ultimate significance." Fr. Spitzer writes: "*Espirit de corps* arises out of the minds and hearts of inspired leaders, and inspired leadership in turn depends upon an internal disposition that allows for commitment, ethics, and team leadership. This essential internal disposition may be termed 'freedom from ego-compulsion.'" Yes, this level is part spiritual. Bo combined a tenacious attitude and actions to serve a better tomorrow that he knew he would never see.

Level 1 Happiness: Immediate Physical Gratification

Level 1 happiness is about us and our physical needs. Bo loved working out for an hour every day as he said, "There are few things in life better than fully expending your self with a good workout, sweat dripping everywhere, and taking a long shower to cool down, getting dressed in clothes that make you feel good, and having a great dinner, perhaps with a glass of good wine." The work out, the sweating, the shower, the clothes that felt good, the dinner, and the good wine are all Level 1 immediate physical gratifications.

Level 1 happiness is personally pleasing, does not last very long, and is felt only by ourselves. We are born with it. When an infant is hungry, wet, tired, or cold, we know about it right away. This level of happiness lasts a few hours, as we each know we will need another meal soon, or we will not be happy!

Level 2 Happiness: Ego Gratification

Level 2 happiness is about ego gratification and generally comes in four forms: achievement, comparative advantage, recognition and popularity, and power and control. Bo had all of them, and the first three (achievement, comparative advantage, and recognition and popularity) gave him the fourth—power and control. Bo knew how to use it for the creation of a better tomorrow. Bo knew the role he was to play as a leader of the University of Michigan football team, and he loved that role. It was because of the responsibility he felt to drive for the highest level of happiness that he could perform in such a strong role. It was not about Bo, though the media and his opponents attempted to make him look to be stubborn and single-minded. It was about what Bo needed to do, to fulfill his mission in life "to develop the greatest young men possible, so they may go out and make an even greater difference in tomorrow."

As competitive as Bo was, he exemplified his passion for a higher level of happiness when asked why he did not coach another year to break Woody Hayes' record for the most wins in the Big Ten Conference. He said, "The number of wins you have in a lifetime does not mean a thing, all they mean is you are old, and you coached a long time."

Level 2 happiness is also related to comparing what others have or have achieved. If you are a competitor, you must have this for a sense of accomplishment. As a destination Level of Happiness, it is a life of comparison that has no long-term happiness, because eventually you will be beat in the comparison game. Level 2 happiness is personally pleasing and lasts longer than Level 1, perhaps as long as a winning season. We gain Level 2 happiness before adolescence, when we begin to see that others may have something we want, or vice versa.

Level 3 Happiness: Making a Contribution

Level 3 is about offering what we have to the benefit of others, the team, the family, the organization. Bo lived a set of values that were clearly in alignment with the "Michigan Family's values," and he took that responsibility very seriously. No one worked harder than Bo did. He was tireless in his effort to build the best young men he could, and he appreciated that he had the vehicle of college football to do that in.

The scheduled 92-hour workweeks during football season would take a toll on everyone, and after defeating a significant opponent there was a natural inclination for all the staff to let up a little in the middle of a long season, especially when the next week's opponent was not of the same caliber. That was when you saw the Level 3 sacrifice come out of Bo. Ask any of his staff what it was like to think you had a "break"! Typically it would be Monday morning at the 8:00 AM Staff Meeting, and you could feel the desire to take a week to recover. Then Bo would push someone's button, usually the hot-tempered Irish line coach Jerry Hanlon, and pretty soon the intensity of the meeting changed drastically and the energy was there to do the job that needed to be done. When was Bo's recovery time? We do not know, but he knew that we needed to be disciplined to delay the gratification after a victory for the possibility of an even greater happiness after a great week of preparation and playing a great game.

Level 3 happiness is all about contributing to others to make them better individually or organizationally. We gain this in adulthood, and as we become parents. We see some young people with this and we marvel at their maturity. We do not see it in some, and we wonder why they lack it. The salaries and bonuses paid to professional athletes were a great concern of Bo's, as they had not achieved this level of adulthood. He feared they would be forever living in a comparison world of those who have more material things than they did. Level 3 happiness lasts longer than Level 2. Some of Bo's greatest Level 3 gratifications came at team reunions, when he could see what the young men he impacted had become, the families they were raising, and the contributions they were making to others and to their communities.

Level 4 Happiness: Being Involved with Something of Ultimate Significance

Level 4, as Fr. Spitzer writes, "is the joy that comes from being involved with something of ultimate significance." Bo lived this level of happiness as his mission "to develop the greatest young men possible, so they may go out and make an even greater difference in tomorrow."

Bo seldom had bad days, because it was never about "today." It was always about a better tomorrow, and he understood his role in making that possible. The media was confused by Bo with his seemingly large ego, yet he wasn't about records, money, or individual accolades. When you begin to understand his Level 4 focus on a better tomorrow, then you can understand why he was, well, the way he was! He had his game plan on developing each of his players to be the best person they could be, and the media wanted stories to make headlines. Bo did not want or need their help in the development of these young men! They wanted a news story for today, but Bo was about what difference they'd make tomorrow!

Giving his players the right values for lifetime decision making was Bo's greatest gift to them and he knew it and they eventually got it, too. The game of football provided this wonderful vehicle for him and he relished it. That is what made leaving Michigan football earlier than he wanted so difficult. Again, it was the delayed gratification of the wins on Saturday that he gave up, at the suggestion of his doctors, to live a longer life and continue to be there to impact new lives and the lives of his former players who called on him daily.

Fritz Seyferth had the opportunity to spend a weekend with Bo late in his life at the National College Football Hall of Fame Dinner, and saw every minute filled with touching as many other lives as Bo could, taking time, only when he had to, to take a nap or to sleep. Two days of catching up with the who's who of college football, former players, and coaches were exemplified when, after the big dinner at which Bo was a featured speaker, they turned the lights out and the emergency lights came on in order for Bo to get his entourage to leave the banquet hall! Bo had told Jamie Morris, one of his players, and the UM Athletic Department staff that had driven down from Ann Arbor for the dinner and were returning that same evening, to meet him at the hotel after the dinner. It was already late in the evening, when as he was leaving the darkened ballroom to meet up with the UM Athletic Department staff who were waiting on him, when he noticed a young man clearing the tables. Bo stopped and asked the young man what high school he went to, what his grades were, what sports did he play, did he want to play football in college, where did he want to go to school. And after he had politely answered each of the questions, Bo shook the young man's hand and said, "Young man, keep that attitude and you are going to do great things."

Level 4 happiness is gained later in life for most, as it takes a level of maturity to see beyond today to a better tomorrow that we can have an impact upon if we invest ourselves in it. Bo honored Levels 1–3 in service of Level 4, to achieve his ultimate level of happiness, which enabled him to say, "How can people say 'I am having a bad day'? How can you have a bad day?"

It was Bo's desire to publicly share his medical battles in this book for the purpose of helping others who are experiencing the same battle with hopes that they might better understand what they are going through and how he faced his challenges. In the end, this book and Bo's battles are worthwhile, not for personal gain, but for the purpose of creating a better tomorrow for others.

Final Overtime

In the third week of October 2006, Coach Schembechler had a frightening episode just before filming his weekly television show. He described it as a spell. "Like my heart was rolling over and over." Although Bo didn't pass out, for 30 seconds he was barely responsive. Suddenly the symptoms passed. Fearing something serious and heart related, the producers of the television show called emergency medical services who arrived on the scene. In typical Bo Schembechler fashion, after having been restored to normalcy, he asked the paramedical team to stand by while they completed the show! After taping the interview, he was walking to the ambulance when he had another episode, which nearly made him unconscious. "It felt like a sinking feeling and as if this might be the end." Once again, fate was with him and his heart returned to its rhythm.

Following an ambulance ride to a local hospital, he was airlifted to the University of Michigan Hospital in Ann Arbor, where he underwent further tests. These confirmed that Bo had suffered a dangerously fast arrhythmia arising from the lower pumping chambers of the heart, known as ventricular tachycardia. This arrhythmia, if sustained, frequently leads to a very irregular and more rapid rhythm called ventricular fibrillation, which usually is fatal. Interrogation of Bo's pacemaker with an electronic device confirmed that he had several episodes of fast ventricular tachycardia, which fortunately did not lead to sudden death. In addition, it was clear that the previous three weeks had seen a worsening in his exercise fatigue and tendency to retain fluid in his legs, signs suggesting his underlying heart muscle was getting weaker.

In considering the possible options, his medical team turned to recent advances in arrhythmia technology to provide assistance. First, to mitigate such a dangerously fast cardiac arrhythmia coming from the lower pumping chambers, he had a defibrillator implanted. This internal pacemaker device is capable of terminating dangerously fast arrhythmias of the heart. If a patient develops such an arrhythmia, a surveillance system in the device "looks" at the arrhythmia and decides whether it is dangerous. If it deems that it is, it quickly paces the heart to try to terminate the arrhythmia. If this doesn't work, the device provides a shock to the electrical system of the heart to erase the abnormal circuit and allow the normal heart rhythm pathways to take over.

In addition to this internal defibrillator, Bo's medical team also implanted a different type of pacemaker. Sometimes, when the heart is very weak, the right pumping chamber of the heart (the right ventricle) and the left pumping chamber of the heart (the left ventricle) don't beat in perfect rhythm. When this happens, some of the efficiencies of the heart's pumping function are lost. Given the fact that Bo's recent symptoms suggested additional weakening of his heart muscle, it made sense to place a biventricular pacemaker to try to perfectly synchronize the pumping actions of both sides of his heart.

After three or four days in the hospital, Bo was able to go home and he felt better. His energy seemed to improve, his attitude stayed focused, and he resumed exercise and other activities, including going to football practice, taping his weekly television show, and doing other radio and TV interviews. While his stamina was not quite what it was prior to the incident, his mental ability, focus, fight, and determination were unwavering.

During Ohio State week, the Wolverines prepared to take on the Ohio State Buckeyes in Columbus, Ohio. Bo was ready to help in the effort in any way he could to support the team. The anticipation for this rivalry game never needs extra hype, but this particular year the attention on this game reached a fever pitch that went far beyond the borders of Ohio and Michigan. For the first time in history, the two teams would meet with perfect records, ranked numbers 1 and 2 in the country.

More than ever, Bo Schembechler wanted to be part of his team. Each day, he went to practice. He gave interviews, spoke on talk shows, was filmed for future documentaries, and fulfilled other functions for either the football program or the university. On Thursday, November 16, he spoke to his doctor and said he was having difficulty sleeping and breathing. When asked to come in to be seen for a visit that day, he deferred to the following day, at which time he knew all the preparation he could provide the Michigan team would be complete. Coach Lloyd Carr had asked if Bo would briefly address the team, which was one of his greatest joys. On that day, he addressed the University of Michigan football team for the final time. He gave them a rousing pep talk before their journey to Columbus, one all on that team would remember for a lifetime.

On the following morning, after conducting a radio interview en route to the television studio, Coach Schembechler collapsed at the studio. Studio personnel immediately initiated CPR, and he was rushed to a local hospital. Assessment of his internal defibrillator confirmed that Bo had had not one but a series of episodes of ventricular fibrillation for which his device successfully brought him back into a regular rhythm. Despite a restored heart rhythm, his heart muscle was not generating adequate blood pressure. During the effort to resuscitate Bo, a special device was placed into his aorta, called an intra-aorta balloon pump, to give further assistance to the heart muscle, but again the blood pressure was inadequate. An emergent cardiac catheterization was performed to evaluate whether there had been a sudden discontinuation of blood through his one remaining bypass graft. The blood flow appeared to be adequate. Careful checks of all possible metabolic causes for heart depression identified no reversal cause for his failing heart muscle. At 11:42 AM on November 17, 2006, Coach Bo Schembechler passed at the age of 77.

In the days that followed Bo Schembechler's death, the true impact that he had on the University of Michigan, Ann Arbor, the State of Michigan, and college athletics throughout the country became increasingly evident. University students held a candlelight vigil on campus the night of his passing. Thousands of well-wishers passed by his body during a public visitation at St. Andrew's Episcopal Church in Ann Arbor. Hundreds of former players and coaches descended on Ann Arbor for a memorial celebration of Bo's life, attended by 15,000 people at Michigan Stadium. In local and national news reports and publications, his life's defining principles and milestones were talked about with uncommon respect, appreciation, and admiration.

What also came to pass in those days after his death was a deepening appreciation for his remarkable medical battle with heart disease over nearly four decades. Colleagues, family, friends, and interested fans began to reflect on his remarkable medical journey. Bo fought his medical foes of coronary heart disease and diabetes with a quiet determination that defied the odds. And as he wanted, he lived his life fully right to the end.

When we step back to consider his life after his first heart attack, at the Rose Bowl on December 31, 1969, we see a man who endured two heart attacks, two coronary bypass operations, years of insulin-dependent diabetes, kidney insufficiency, diabetic neuropathy, arthritis, gout, two pacemakers, an arrhythmia ablation, heart failure and fought the war against heart disease for four decades!

Epilogue

In the days following Bo's passing, friends and members of the media wrote and spoke about Bo's life, coaching, and his fight to survive. Just a few representative reflections are included here.

Mitch Albom, *Detroit Free Press*—The old man's voice will never be silenced. And yet the man himself is gone, done in by the very organ that truly defined him: his heart. It was tragic and sudden and awful and shocking, and it was exactly the way we knew it would happen. Bo told me, "I will die one day from a bad heart." As usual, the old man was right. We should have seen it coming. Thirty-seven years ago, he was walking up a hill in Pasadena, California, alone, in the dark, and he felt a stabbing pain and he grabbed a tree to hold himself up. He was nearly 40 then, but that incident—the night before his first Rose Bowl—was his first heart attack. Friday's incident, when he was 77—the day before the biggest Michigan–Ohio State game ever—was his last. In between there were too many surgeries, procedures, EKGs, a pacemaker, too many scary rushes to the hospital with everyone thinking, "Is this it?" But Bo came back from them all. Sooner or later, there he was, Michigan's Lazarus, in a natty sports coat with a maize-and-blue tie, and he'd be barking his same old bark and telling people he was a medical miracle, and, well, after awhile, you just figured he could straight-arm anything, even mortality.

But if death doesn't get you at the shoulders it will get you at the knees, if not by the front, then from behind. And so, during a taping Friday morning of his weekly television show on Channel 7, doing the thing he liked second-best, talking about football—coaching it always would be No. 1—death tried blindsiding Bo once more. And this time, the only time, it took him down.

Erik Smith, ABC News—I walked by and he said, "Hey, kid." I turned around. He said, "I hear you have joined the club." I said, "What club?" He said, "The Zipper Club." I said, "What are you talking about?" He said, "You got a zipper in your chest now, don't you?" I said, "That club."

So I am a proud member of the Zipper Club. I don't know if Bo invented that phrase, but it stuck. He had two major bypass operations and two heart attacks and he did have a health scare last month right here at Channel 7. Bo and I are in the Zipper Club!

Bo had tremendous care at the University of Michigan Hospital as well and we talked about the fund-raising that he did for cancer research there. The doctors at that hospital and that hospital system loved Bo Schembechler. They appreciated him. They have provided him with wonderful, wonderful care over the years including the most recent episode prior to today ... He ended up at another local hospital but he needed to get to the University of Michigan because they know his history. He had just received that pacemaker and heart defibrillator combined into one.

**Michael Rosenberg, *Detroit Free Press*—He had said it with so much conviction—"I'm not gonna die"—that it was hard to doubt him, despite all the evidence. Isn't that the strangest thing? He had dodged death for so many years, it was like he was immune to it. Bo Schembechler might be the only person ever to die shockingly after a 37-year battle with heart trouble.

Jo-Ann Barnas, *Akron Beacon Journal*—Three months ago, Schembechler paid a visit to his hometown in Ohio and spoke frankly about his health problems. "I have had two heart attacks and two open-heart surgeries," Schembechler told the *Akron Beacon Journal*. "I am a diabetic. I have a pacemaker. At the medical complex at Michigan, they say it is a miracle I am alive. And I had fried chicken for lunch!"

Bob Wojnowski, *Detroit News*—He went as far as he could go, farther than many doctors long expected, and then he could go no farther. To the very day his damaged heart finally stopped working, Bo Schembechler never stopped using it, every flawed ounce of it. Schembechler, who won more games than any coach in Michigan history before retiring in 1989, squeezed everything he could out of his scarred chest, operated on four times in 36 years. Schembechler often laughed that he'd cheated death for years, ever since he suffered a heart attack on the eve of the 1970 Rose Bowl, but a growing reality could not be avoided. Schembechler had three mantras he never relinquished. He preached "The team, the team, the team." He promised, "Those who stay will be champions." And he said, "What the mind can conceive and believe, the body can achieve." All were true to the end, all but the last. The mind was alive, but the body was spent. A giant is gone, beaten by an old nemesis he was weary of fighting.

Lynn Henning, *Detroit News*—He was 77 years old, a blessedly lengthy life for a man who had been staring down the barrel of coronary artery disease since he was 40.

Angelique Chengelis, *Detroit News*—A few weeks ago, when Bo had recovered from a health scare, he was at the Channel 7 studios to tape *Big Ten Ticket*. Bo had agreed to meet with me that day. He came over, hugged me, kissed me on the cheek, and went about his preparations for the show. Afterward, we talked. He talked about cheating death. About being in the ambulance, knowing he was not in good shape and looking up at his wife, Cathy, and thinking he could not leave now. He joked he had the "Cadillac" of heart mechanisms in his chest, a combination defibrillator/pacemaker. And in a flashback to that day in southern California, I asked him if he could feel the device, and if it gave him any discomfort. Bo opened the left side of his jacket and he told me to put my hand on his chest. I put my hand over his heart and was surprised how large the device was. He didn't care. It was keeping him alive, and that's all that mattered.

Jim Carty, *Ann Arbor News*—Afterward, at the 1970 Rose Bowl, Schembechler suffered his first heart attack. "I'll never forget that, when they came to tell us at 11 AM that Bo had had a heart attack," (former player Dick) Caldorazzo said. "They said, 'He's fine, don't worry about it,' but I never saw so many guys in shock. Half the team was crying, half the team was in shock. It wasn't because we were without a coach. It was because we really lost somebody who was like a father to us. I told Bo that if they'd only let us see him, if we knew he was OK, it would have been different. A lot of us felt he might have been gone." "He just wouldn't slow down," (former player Garvie) Craw said

Friday, with touches of both sadness and anger in his voice. "He just wouldn't say no to anybody," the former fullback said. "I asked him, 'Bo, just do two less things this week so you can be around with us next spring.' He considered it his responsibility. He was old school. It was part of what made Bo. We're going to miss that guy."

Christina Hildreth, *Michigan Daily*—On October 20, 2006 he was taping the show *Big Ten Ticket* at WXYZ studios in Southfield when he collapsed on the set. He spent four days in the hospital, but it didn't seem to dampen his spirits. History English Prof. John Bacon said Bo often gave the nurses a hard time. Two days after the operation, Bacon said, a nurse checked in on the man who had come to embody Michigan football. She asked him how much he weighed. He responded firmly: "Young lady, I weigh 195 pounds of blue twisted steel."

Drew Sharp, *Detroit Free Press*—He devoured the quest for victory, just ate it up. It wasn't about winning, but the discipline and work ethic demanded to reach that plateau. And although the ravishes of a decades-long battle with heart disease coupled with complications from diabetes inevitably quieted that indomitable spirit, Bo was truly the Victor in his toughest fight. He beat heart disease because he never let it beat him. He attacked it like he did a vulnerable defensive line. He survived more than 36 years after suffering that first heart attack right before his first Rose Bowl as Michigan's head coach on New Year's Eve 1969. If heart disease were a football opponent, today it's catching its breath, steadying its legs and wiping its brow, thoroughly exhausted from a knockdown, dragged-out fight to the finish. And that's how Bo went into every Saturday. You may beat him, but you'll walk away wearing the bruises from a backroom brawl. On Friday, doctors called it a "testament to his will" that he defied medical logic for as long as he did, but he'll be remembered for far more than just winning football games. And that's an enduring testament to his humanity.

Dawn Jones, ABC 12 News—Bo Schembechler fought a courageous battle against heart disease and diabetes for nearly 40 years. For the past five years, Dr. Kim Eagle was Bo's personal physician. Dr. Eagle spoke at today's press conference about the man he called one of his "most courageous patients. He has defied all odds in his survival with really remarkably bad heart disease. Even in the past six to nine months when we worked together to try to deal with a failing heart pump and issues with his electrical system, he was absolutely determined to continue his battle to win every day to meet the next possibility."

Two Remarkable and Wonderful Eulogies

Thank you to Coach Bobby Knight and author/media talent Mitch Albom for permission to share their eulogies. They are special and we hope you enjoy them.

Bo and Bobby Knight were at Ohio State together when Bo was an assistant to Woody Hayes and Bobby Knight was on the OSU basketball team. Their friendship grew from that time on. This eulogy was in longhand on hotel stationery and was faxed to be read at Bo's memorial service, as Coach Knight was traveling with the Texas Tech basketball team. Bo once called Bobby Knight his "best friend in coaching."

Coach Bobby Knight's Eulogy of Bo—During those last moments before eternal peace came to him, I'm sure Bo was thinking of all the people, family, and friends who had been close to him during his lifetime. Most of all, I'd bet he was thinking of Cathy who, for the last 13 years, has exposed him to places that he didn't even know existed. Yet, during those last moments, I also believe that he looked the grim reaper right in the eye and said, "You son-of-a-bitch, you've been trying to get me since that first heart attack in 1970 and I've beaten your ass for 36 years!"

I know that every player who has ever played for Bo, if asked what teacher in his educational experience had taught him the most about success in life ... the answer, without exception, would be Bo.

Now, I'd like to take just a moment to address the almighty God; I don't know if you've met and talked to Bo yet or not but, I'm sure that in the short time he's been with you he has found that in some areas your people up there are throwing too many passes and not running enough, while, in other places, there is some sloppy blocking and tackling going on. Now my advice, God, would be that you immediately put him in charge of heavenly organization and discipline. He's made things far better everywhere he's been and I know he'll do the same for you. One other thing now, God, don't even ask him a question that you don't want an honest answer to. He might seem a little bit opinionated at first ... just keep in mind that he's right one hell of a lot more than he's ever wrong.

Well, God, that's about it. We've sent you the best we've ever had. Listen to him, trust him completely, and don't try to change him. I've never seen a coach of any sport who was better than Bo. Nor have I ever had a friend that I cherished more.

Mitch Albom's Eulogy of Bo—At Bo's funeral at St. Andrew's Episcopal Church, his friend and *Detroit Free Press* columnist read his letter of recommendation for Coach Schembechler.

Dear God—

By now, you have already received Bo Schembechler, and although it's only been a couple of days, you may have noticed he is not your typical incoming freshman. He's brasher than most. He's more courageous than most. He's funnier than most. And the only thing he's ever been late for was you, and that's because he fought the weak heart you gave him longer than anyone down here had a right to expect. Excuse his tardiness. Maybe it's our fault. We didn't want to let him go. And since Bo worked most of his life at universities, where letters of recommendation are required for admittance, on the off chance that heaven works the same way, please consider the following such a recommendation letter.

First, we can only imagine that Bo arrived through your pearly gates and, upon saying hello, asked for the nearest television set. He meant no disrespect. You see, he coached a little game down here called football. He did more than coach it. He shaped it. He became part of its fabric. Saturdays in the fall were a religion for him, much like Sundays are for, well, you. He loved his flock the way you love yours. It's just that his wore pads or carried clipboards and dressed in the same two colors every day. He was just thinking of them when he arrived up there, that's all. You can't blame him for that.

And if he kicked over the TV set somewhere around 6:30 on Saturday, well, let's just say if you have a special cloud for Ohio Staters, you probably don't want Bo there.

Now, there are some things we should confess to you about Bo. He wasn't perfect. He had a temper. And he used your name once or twice—and maybe not the way you intended it. But it was always to make a point, trying to get someone to behave the right way, trying to stand on principle.

You see, Bo believed in principle. He believed in honesty, in not cheating or stealing, and in honoring his elders—the very things you once carved into tablets. He learned these principles from his parents in Ohio, and he passed them on to his sons in Michigan—all his sons—the ones who shared his name and the thousands of others who shared his locker room.

By the way, on the subject of names, you're fortunate, God, that you don't have a last name, because Bo would probably call you by it. He did that to us down here. He loved to throw his arm around us and put his meaty grip on our necks and toss us a friendly insult or two. Don't count this against him. Being teased by Bo was one of the great joys of our lives. Once, one of his players actually made a mistake on purpose, and when Bo demanded to know why, the guy said he just wanted to hear Bo yell at him.

In that way, God, he was a little like you. Because he taught, because he moved people, because he made us richer for coming in contact with him, because he turned boys into men and men into better men, sometimes, as with you, we just wanted to hear his voice, even if the voice was angry, even if his answer was no. He made us feel alive. That's why we never wanted him to die. We've been walking around telling ourselves "it was his time," but it was not his time. Not in a hospital on a Friday.

Bo's time was patrolling the sidelines on chilly autumn afternoons. His time was with his wife and his children and his grandchildren. His time was looking up from his desk and seeing a former player poke his head in and surprise him. His time was having a juicy hamburger put in front of him with nobody around to tell him he shouldn't eat it.

Those were his times, God.

But we know you know that.

We can give Bo high marks in the family department, God. He loved his first wife, Millie, and took her three sons under his wing. He loved his youngest boy, Shemy, and when Shemy was born, the nurse put him right next to the newborn daughter of one of his players, Garvie Craw, and Bo and Garvie stood side by side at the glass, and Bo said, "Keep your daughter away from him ..." That had to be your doing, right, God? Who else could set up a line like that?

When Millie was called to you, Bo honored her memory, raising more money to fight the disease that took her than any army could do.

Maybe because of that, you gave him a gift, God, when you sent him his second wife, Cathy. You gave wings to his dormant heart, and everyone here knows that Cathy gave us extra years with Bo. You live better when you love, and Bo lived better in love than he ever would have alone.

As for accommodations, well, Bo won't need much up there, God, because he was never a things guy. He began at Michigan with a folding chair and a clothes hook and if you want to give him that again—save the fancy stuff for the Pac Ten coaches—well, he won't mind.

But please, God, surround him with people.

Because the thing you should know about Glenn Schembechler, and the real reason he was late for his arrival up there, is that he was busy with people down here on earth. He was busy molding them and scolding them, busy visiting them in hospitals, busy counseling their children, busy flying across the country to support their banquets, busy, once, even walking a former player to a jailhouse door, encouraging him to stay strong. It takes time to give so much, God. It takes time to be there for so many people. Bo filled the unforgiving minute with sixty seconds' worth of distance run, just like that poem says, but he ran it more for others than himself.

And isn't that sort of the golden rule, God? Isn't that the highest recommendation we can offer?

So please accept this letter as the strongest of endorsements. Bo will make heaven a livelier place, a more passionate place, and if the angels are looking to get a little game going, you could do worse than to put him in charge.

But please consider this request: let Bo come back to us now and then. Not in body. But in heart, in mind. Let us hear the gruff voice once in a while, yelling at us to block harder or to tackle lower. Let us feel that big paw around our shoulders when it's cold and we are alone. Let us see that crinkling smile and hear that hearty laugh when we drop into our dreams at night.

And let him yell at us now and again, when we aren't living up to his standards, because living up to his standards is amongst the finest things we'll ever do.

Take care of him, God. And if you have such things up there, would you please give him a whistle? He'll know what to do with it.

Signed,

The people on earth who have been touched by Bo Schembechler, and who are far, far, too numerous to mention.

Acknowledgments

This book was made possible by Bo's tireless efforts to ensure tomorrow will be better than today for those who battle cardiovascular disease as he did and by all those who cared so deeply about this remarkable man. His energy behind this book did not make its publishing an option, it was an obligation. First, the sacrifice of the spouses of authors who read more rough text than anyone should have to … Cathy Schembechler, Lynn Seyferth, and Darlene Eagle.

The medical information provided alongside Bo Schembechler's account of fighting cardiovascular disease and diabetes was garnered from a team that Bo recruited and selected to care for him. These include the faculty and staff of the University of Michigan Cardiovascular Center and its Preventive Cardiology programs, St. Joseph Mercy Hospital and its Michigan Heart and Vascular Institute, as well as materials from the American Heart Association, National Institutes of Health, American Diabetes Association, and from scientific guidelines published by the American College of Cardiology/American Heart Association. The medical summaries and recommendations that accompany Bo Schembechler's story are not meant to be either exhaustive or necessarily complete. The authors do not claim ownership for their substance or language. However, the summaries provide the lay audience a thumbnail sketch of the medical issues faced by Coach Schembechler and the manner in which he and his care team chose to attack those problems. The authors of the book are indebted to all of the above noted entities for their contributions and publicly distributed materials that went into the creation of *The Heart of a Champion.* We are especially indebted to Bo Schembechler and his wife Cathy and his family for their desire to tell his story.

To those who helped pull all the pieces together, without whom this book would not have been possible: Lisa Hackbarth, Jeanna Cooper, Gary Bondie, John Bacon, Jim Edwards, Skip DeWall, Mary Passink, Shemy & Meghan Schembechler, Jim Stanley M.D., Mel Rubenfire M.D., Kathy Rhodes, Rich Prager M.D., Jeff Sanfield M.D., David Pinsky M.D., Greg Kinney, Mitch Albom, Jim & Robbie Brandstatter, Per Kjeldsen, and the leader of the team Cathy Schembechler.

And to those who touched Bo's life as much as he touched theirs and contributed greatly to the content of this book: Lloyd Carr, Gary Moeller, Jerry Hanlon, Rudy Reichert M.D., Otto Gago M.D., Jon Falk, Lynn Koch, Alex Agase, President Jerry Ford, Bobby Knight, and Dan Ewald.

Thank you to each for being a team in Bo's truest sense of the word. Your efforts were amazing, and you made it fun, energizing, and very rewarding to be on your team …

About This Book

Because his medical story was so unique and so inspiring, Bo had agreed to work with his most recent cardiologist Kim Eagle and former player and dear friend Fritz Seyferth to create this book in late 2005. In typical Bo fashion, he hesitated to bring attention to his own life or medical circumstances. As his medical battles continued, however, and with precious time near the end for reflection, he began to understand that the lessons he'd learned through this medical journey might help others facing similar challenges. This was his motivation. If he could help you, the reader, then he would have been a successful coach, again!

With his coauthors, he agreed that all of their proceeds emanating from the sale of the book would be placed in the "Bo Schembechler's Heart of a Champion Fund" at the University of Michigan's Cardiovascular Center. The fund would be invested in cardiovascular research with hopes that new observations in prevention, diagnosis, and treatment of cardiovascular disease will help others in the same way that Bo benefited from a series of medical and surgical advances. Bo loved the idea that he might be able to facilitate research breakthroughs that would ultimately help each of us "win" in our own medical battles, just as he had for so long.

As Cathy Schembechler stated in her support of the Bo Schembechler Heart of a Champion Fund: "Advances in medicine and science gave Bo years that all who loved and respected him so much appreciated. And now we need to continue those remarkable advances to give others more time with their loved ones, who like Bo made a difference in the world every extra day he had."

Bo Schembechler defied all odds in his medical battle against cardiovascular disease. His medical success was predicated on discipline, trust, hard work, the setting of clear goals, terrific coordination of his caregivers and medications, steadily taking advantage of scientific break-throughs in diagnosis and treatment, and an attitude of never-ending desire to live each and every day to the full-est. Like his success in football, his medical success was realized one day at a time.

What the mind and scientific advances can conceive and believe, the person and their care team can achieve!

God bless you, Bo.

Index

Pictured on the back cover are members of Bo's team *(left to right):* Fritz Seyferth, Dr. Eric Good, Dr. Eva Feldman, Mary Passink, Dr. Fred Morady, Dr. Otto Gago, Dr. Jeff Sanfield, Cathy Schembechler, Dr. Kim Eagle, Dr. Rudy Reichert, Dr. Dennis Wahr, Dr. Jim Stanley, Dr. Jim Carpenter, Dr. Dave Fox, and Dr. Hakan Oral.